THE ROCK CARLING FELLOWSHIP

1977

Research in medicine

PROBLEMS AND PROSPECTS

THE ROCK CARLING FELLOWSHIP

1977

RESEARCH IN MEDICINE

PROBLEMS AND PROSPECTS

Sir Andrew Watt Kay

THE NUFFIELD
PROVINCIAL HOSPITALS TRUST
1977

Published by the
Nuffield Provincial Hospitals Trust
3 Prince Albert Road, London NW1 7SP

ISBN 0 900574 27 5

Designed by Bernard Crossland
PRINTED IN GREAT BRITAIN BY
BURGESS & SON (ABINGDON) LTD
ABINGDON, OXFORDSHIRE

The Rock Carling Fellowship
was founded as an annual memorial
to the late Sir Ernest Rock Carling,
for many years a Governing Trustee
of the Nuffield Provincial Hospitals Trust
and Chairman of the Trust's Medical
Advisory Committee

Each holder of the fellowship
will seek to review in a monograph
the state of knowledge and activity
in one of the fields in which Sir Ernest
had been particularly interested and which
is within the purposes of the Trust.
The arrangements provide that the
monograph will be introduced by a
public lecture to be given at
a recognized medical teaching centre
in the United Kingdom

CONTENTS

PREFACE

My predecessors elected to the Rock Carling Fellowship have all regarded this as a great honour. For me it has a particular significance, and this for three reasons. First, my election to this Fellowship takes place exactly one hundred years after the birth of Ernest Rock Carling. Secondly, although his interests and contributions extended beyond the realms of surgery, Rock Carling was one of the leading surgeons of his day and retired from the Westminster Hospital in the same year (1942) in which I proudly changed my title from 'Dr' to 'Mr' on gaining the FRCS diploma; I am grateful for this opportunity to pay my small tribute to one who played his part in moulding the progress of surgery in this country. To be elected to the Fellowship when a Trustee of the Nuffield Provincial Hospitals Trust is intriguing, but I would hasten to add that the Trustees establish a special Panel with the responsibility for choosing the subject and electing the Fellow: although the Trustees must give formal approval, the Panel does not include any of the Trustees! I agreed to make the Trustees' approval unanimous.

The subject allocated to me was broadly, 'The future of medical research'. On contemplating this formidable task it seemed to me that the even tenor of progress in medical research over the past fifty years had been disturbed by a series of new influences, many of which had occurred in the course of the past decade. And so, in my view, any attempt to peer into the future would require a prior attempt to assess the impact and probable outcome of these new factors. It is for this reason that I have selected the title 'Problems and Prospects in Medical Research'.

An underlying theme is the importance of maintaining a balance among the several forms of research related to medicine. The preservation of balance in the natural world confronts us constantly and we should now know that nature abhors massive changes in a positive or negative direction, but we tend to be so involved in the affairs of the present that this lesson is not taken to heart. Biomedical research, clinical research, and research directed towards improving the health services comprise a unity, and among these three a reasonable balance should be preserved, change monitored, and major deviations corrected; they are interdependent and so, for example, advances on the biomedical front will call for health services research, and progress in the latter will call for more biomedical research. This is no time for controversy and debate on the relative merits and boundaries of the several arms of research in medicine; it is no time to conceive or harbour antagonisms which will only militate against progress. This is a time for scientists, doctors, sociologists, economists, behavioural scientists, and others to work together on major problems, study these with accepted methodology, and advocate change on the basis of sound evidence; this will be the strongest armour against the arrows of bureaucracy.

The Rothschild proposals, confirmed in the White Paper on *The Framework for Government Research and Development*, have had a profound impact on medical research. While some would regard this influence as entirely harmful, it contains the seeds which may yield good fruit. The health departments have been given the challenge of establishing research agencies which could be effective in influencing decision making and in promoting a better health service. My own conviction that a Chief Scientist Organization should ensure the close articulation of research management, the executive department, and the scientific community is my excuse for describing at some length the establishment of the CSO within the Scottish Home and Health Department.

Medical science has not escaped the general reaction against science and technology which has gained momentum during the past decade. Perhaps society has expected too much; perhaps society has become too anxious about the outcome of some scientific researches because these have been excessively underlined by the mass media. In any event there has been a movement against a continuing search for knowledge and this has been accompanied by a growing demand for studies which have clear practical objectives. Some movement in this direction is not without merit and it must be acknowledged that the patronage of research is now provided by society to whom researchers must be accountable.

One very important aspect of accountability is to communicate clearly, honestly, and with full explanation of intent to our patrons. The responsibility of reversing an unmistakable loss of confidence in the value and effectiveness of science rests with the scientific community.

Progress in research depends to a large extent on the recruitment of good scientists and at the present time several influences are affecting this adversely. These include increasingly inflexible training programmes for medical graduates, financial disincentives, nil growth rates in research budgets, and the severe financial constraints now placed on our universities which are the seed-beds for future research workers.

These are among the problems to be considered before I seek the help of my crystal ball to speculate on future trends in medical research.

This essay includes few tables and no figures, graphs, or statistics; many publications—not a few sponsored by the Nuffield Provincial Hospitals Trust—provide the background information on which it is based. References are provided throughout the text for those who would wish to study in greater depth any aspect of the subject which may arouse their interest and enthusiasm.

There have been remarkable advances in medicine and greater advances are to come. Since the beginning of time, man's search for happiness has been nullified by the unrelenting shadow of disease and suffering. Shelley, with the poet's eye, saw signs of the dawn, but this was slow to break and only in the past two centuries has the bright sun of achievement begun to disperse the darkness which surrounds the great personal fear of every man: ill health and physical pain.

> Even where the milder zone afforded man
> A seeming shelter, yet contagion there,
> Blighted his being with unnumbered ills,
> Spread like a quenchless fire; nor truth availed
> Till late to arrest its progress, or create
> The peace which first in bloodless victory waved
> Her snowy standard o'er this favoured clime.
> . . . Happiness
> And Science dawn though late upon the earth; . . .

Preface

History will surely record this century as forever memorable in that the storehouses of Nature, laid open by science and research, have bestowed on man blessings which transcend even his most fanciful longings and speculations. Material progress is evidenced by the first tentative excursions into outer space, the development of atomic power, and the impact of electronics on every aspect of human existence. Social advancement is manifest in the great improvement in the general standard of living, and in the progressive diffusion of education. Remarkable though they are, the fruits of these achievements may not compare with the diminution in physical suffering which has followed in the wake of scientific advances in medicine and which humanity has waited generations to see. The future holds exciting prospects which will be enhanced provided that support for scientific research is maintained, that we can ensure movement in the right directions, and that medical research in particular is organized in an increasingly effective manner.

ACKNOWLEDGEMENTS

I am grateful to the many friends and colleagues who have educated and stimulated me through the years and so provided any background I may have on research related to medicine; in particular I would like to thank Dr Michael Ashley-Miller with whom I have had many valuable discussions, but I would emphasize that I accept full responsibility for the views expressed in this essay. I am indebted to my friend Gordon McLachlan who read the draft and gave me valuable advice. My most sincere thanks go to my secretary, Miss Lilian Barron, who did all the typing in her usual willing and meticulous fashion. Finally, I am especially grateful to my best friend, my wife, for her understanding tolerance of my hasty withdrawal to the study after dinner on most evenings during the past few months.

I

Prelude to Rothschild

A relationship between science and society, and the concept of research as a social activity, seems to be regarded by many as a development in our time. There is little doubt that there has been a growing realization of the impact of scientific research on the needs and demands of society, but it is of interest that more than half of the problems handled by the Royal Society in the first thirty years after its establishment in 1662 were prompted by the practical needs of public use: Evelyn investigated and campaigned against the smoke which polluted the air of London; Sir William Petty published a treatise on taxes and contributions; at about this time too William Harvey was exhorting medical scientists to advance knowledge by way of experiment and to bear in mind the importance of developing their contribution to society. It is likely, however, that while scientists were aware of their responsibilities, society had not at that time any real awareness of the activities of the scientists; this is not surprising when one considers that the research worker of that day had to work entirely on his own with very simple facilities, requiring at most the encouragement and financial support of an interested patron. Today research is a team affair which often calls for the involvement of several disciplines and demands financial support beyond the gift of individual patronage. By the turn of the century it was apparent that research required public funding and a national organization both for its promotion and to satisfy public requirements.

State support of medical research in the United Kingdom began with the introduction of the National Insurance Act in 1911. Each insured person contributed the equivalent of one penny per week, the sum being allocated for the purposes of research in relation to health. The first Medical Research Committee was formed with a budget of £53,000 in 1913 to undertake research 'into any disease to which insured persons are subject'. This budget remained unchanged until after the First World War. When the end of the war was in sight a committee was formed, under the chairmanship of Lord Haldane to review the machinery of government. The *Report on the Machinery of Government* (Cd 9230, 14 December 1918) distinguished between the intelligence and research work which should be done by departments themselves, and the work which should be done in a general research organization (the prototype of the research council), and emphasized that the relation was a problem in *correlation* rather than in *demarcation*. To ensure that departments would not suppress research which was politically inconvenient, the general research organization was to be placed under the Lord President who would be 'immune from any suspicion of being biased by administrative consideration against the application of research'. Emphasis was placed on making new contributions to knowledge but this was seen as coming from work on the problems put to the general research organization by industry and the departments. However the Addison memorandum of 1919 (1) clearly recognized the error of restricting a research organization's activities to work solely on practical programmes related to current interests:

> it has already been found in many cases that an inquiry started with a purely practical purpose has led scientific men into new inquiries, resulting in fresh discoveries which have been valuable for purposes quite distinct from the solution of the original problem. It has been found equally that the solution of a particular problem has often come unexpectedly from scientific work in some other direction that would have been thought at first sight to be wholly remote from it . . . accordingly, any body of men engaged upon scientific research in medicine, or in any other field, should be given the widest possible freedom to make their new discoveries.

This memorandum, which influenced government policy in Britain for the next half century, led to the incorporation of the Medical Research Council (MRC) under its present title in 1920. Encouraged by Addison's reasoned argument the Council supported research which promised advances in medical and biological knowledge even if the application of that knowledge was not immediately obvious. Again, in deploying its resources it sought out good scientists working in good intellectual environments: universities, selected hospitals, medical practice, and in its own establishments. As this mechanism evolved, an excellent relationship was established between the organization and members of the scientific community; the latter were not administered and were regarded as people rather than personnel. The view has been expressed that the relationship was 'too cosy'; I believe that the climate provided the proper nourishment for research and for researchers. Other developed countries were evolving their own central research organizations and the fact that many took the MRC as a model is an indication of its efficiency and of its success in fulfilling its main objectives: the creation and maintenance of a cadre of good researchers, and the advancement of knowledge in the medical and biological fields.

A second objective of a central research organization is to be responsive to the needs of society which, in turn, demands the forging of adequate links with government. In his Harveian Oration in 1962 Sir Harold Himsworth (2), Secretary of the Medical Research Council, showed his perceptive appreciation of this requirement:

> here scientific considerations are only part of the problem. The relative needs for different types of knowledge, the economic background, social planning, and the ethos of the particular society, all require to be taken into account. All these are political considerations, and at this level political considerations become expert matters in their own right. Further, the resources available, in intellect if not in material are never likely to satisfy all the diversity of needs and interests as conceived by the partisans of each at any particular moment. Considered choices have to be made, and it is the task of general scientific policy to make these. A balance has to be struck between the needs, desires, and resources of a particular society and the relative opportunity, feasibility, and consequences of the various opportunities for developing knowledge that present. It is here that the skills of the politician and the scientist must fuse. Neither can solve these problems alone. Only on a basis of mutual co-operation and respect can they be approached. That such is possible my own experience gives me confidence.

I have personal experience that this was not merely wishful thinking and that the pursuit of the objective was evolving through the next few years.

While a member of the Medical Research Council (1967–71) I recall Council giving further consideration in broad terms to the organization required to support research related to human health. It was decided that four main conditions were mandatory. First, the integral part played by medical research in the total body of research in the natural and social sciences must be taken fully into account at the administrative as well as at the laboratory level. Secondly, research workers and organizations needed to maintain close contact with all those professions and government departments—in particular the medical profession and the health departments—in order to make full use of knowledge in the Council's field of responsibility. Thirdly, the assessment of scientific feasibility, the formulation of scientific aspects of policy and the judgement of scientific proposals and their results can best be undertaken by those with adequate scientific experience. Finally, no artificial division should be allowed to develop between research in the biomedical field and research in the field of health services—between long-term strategic work and short-term tactical investigations. This was evidence of a growing appreciation of the need to develop increasingly close collaboration with the object of ensuring the maintenance of this country's scientific capability together with the application of that capability. There was also a realization at this time of the importance of interdependence between the areas of work of the different research councils; for example, the need to collaborate with the SSRC in order to tackle the challenges facing the social aspects of medicine. It is also worthy of note that MRC activities have always included the promotion of short-term investigations into questions of immediate practical relevance and in my time on Council a growing number of initiatives had been taken in promoting research aimed at particular objectives, not a few of which took into account social need as well as scientific feasibility. The health departments had an input to Council by the presence of the two chief medical officers, and to the clinical and biological research boards through health department nominees. I will discuss later the adequacy of this input, but here it is sufficient to say that a partnership between the research councils and the executive departments was evolving. This was the scene as I saw it prior to the publication of the Rothschild/Dainton proposals in November 1971. Was it necessary or even wise to interfere with this evolving process by creating a major change at a single stroke? I will endeavour in later pages to give at least part answer; in general terms, I believe that major reorganization should be undergone about as often as radical surgery! In these days we tend to meet any new crisis by reorganizing and, in my own experience, it is a magnificent method for creating the illusion of progress while producing confusion, inefficiency, and demoralization.

The introduction of the National Health Service in 1948 coupled with the remarkable progress of scientific medicine in the intervening years, encouraged Parliament to provide increasing financial support so that by 1970 the combined research budget of the MRC and the health departments exceeded £30 million, this sum being more than doubled if other sources of research money are taken into account.

When one considers that this considerable financial support of medical research represented no more than 5 per cent of total government expenditure on research it is not suprising that the state and the public wished to be involved in the choice of the objectives for which the money was being provided. And so the concept grew that it was important to make science a more effective and powerful tool for solving the nation's problems; in our context this means that it became important to consider how medical research can most effectively be organized to resolve major health problems. The growing demand for stricter supervision in medical research was further stimulated by the fact that recent advances in medical science had begun to raise very uncomfortable questions for political decision. The public, gaining 'information' through the mass media, became concerned about the implications of organ transplantation, the determination of the point of death, and the fear that the thalidomide incident might be the forerunner of other drug disasters.

The government of the day had been reviewing the functions of its departments with the aim of ensuring that wherever possible responsibility and accountability were clearly defined and allocated. This review included departmental activities in the field of research and development and as part of this process the government commissioned a report from Lord Rothschild and, in addition, sought advice through the Council for Scientific Policy on the most effective arrangements for organizing and supporting pure and applied scientific research. It is of some interest that the Haldane Report gave no mention of 'pure' as distinct from 'applied' research, nor did it hint that there was any conflict between them.

2

The Rothschild proposals

In the White Paper on *The Reorganisation of Central Government* (Cmnd 4506) it was indicated that all ministers would review the functions of their departments and that this review would include departmental activities in the field of research and development. As part of this exercise the Government commissioned a report from Lord Rothschild on *Government Research and Development*. In addition, they sought advice through the Council for Scientific Policy and this was formulated by a Working Group under the chairmanship of Sir Frederick Dainton. The outcome was a Green Paper *A Framework for Government Research and Development* in November 1971 which contained the two separate reports preceded by a memorandum by the Government.

Rothschild recommended a clear separation of responsibilities between the MRC (responsible for biomedical research) and the health departments (responsible for research planned to improve the health services). In his opinion these were two different kinds of research: biomedical research has as its product an increased knowledge; health service research has as its objective a practical application which from now on should be arranged on a customer/contractor basis—the customer determining what he requires, the contractor doing the work and the customer paying the fee. It should be noted that at this time the MRC was responsible for a recognizable amount of 'applied research' and had been managing this efficiently. However, Lord Rothschild maintained that 'this work had and has no customer to commission and approve it. This is wrong. However distinguished, intelligent, and practical scientists may be, they cannot be so well qualified to decide what the needs of the nation are, and their priorities, as those responsible for ensuring that those needs are met. This is why applied R & D must have a customer', whose role he proceeded to describe in some detail. The fact that the Ministry of Defence had employed this principle for some time in commissioning weapons and tanks was regarded as a sufficient reason for recommending that the health departments should commission biomedical research relevant to their needs: the success, or otherwise, of this translation is discussed later. In the introductory memorandum by the Government the following words appear: 'the Government note that the report of the Council for Scientific Policy is not at variance with this principle'. The truth in these words rests in the fact that the Dainton report at no point mentions the customer/contractor principle. In further support of his argument that applied research and development must be done on a customer/contractor basis Rothschild conceded that chance observations during basic research may occasionally be of importance (presumably such trivia as the discovery of X-rays and penicillin come into this category) but he considered that 'the country's needs are not so trivial as to be left to the mercies of a form of scientific roulette, with many more than the conventional 37 numbers on which the ball may land'. As we shall see, good has come from the Rothschild report, but his advocacy of the customer/contractor principle lacked moderation. It suggested inspiration-to-order and the sacrifice of the freedom of research workers to the wishes of customers who may or may not be sufficiently well informed to define their needs.

Dainton, on the other hand, considered that the growing crisis was not related to the structure of scientific research in Britain, which had been notably successful, but recognized that the departments should play their part in the formulation of scientific policy and, on the other hand, that science could minimize the ignorance of decision-makers. This report provided a reasoned argument indicating that whatever organization was ultimately adopted to manage research and development it should be one that unifies rather than separates scientific activity; one in which the definition of the scientific work would be in the hands of scientists; one which would retain a closer association with the education and training of scientists for the future. This was essentially a confirmation of the research council principle, to which Dainton added the essential qualification that the views and needs of departments, of industry and of professional users should be expressed at all levels, 'as much to those at the bench as to the policy makers'. The report strongly urged that any changes should take the form of a natural evolution from the existing system—as opposed to drastic changes—and that they should combine the very considerable advantages that the existing system has for individual scientists, for scientific organizations and for the universities, with greater flexibility and an improved capacity for service to government departments and to the community.

The Dainton proposals would have been largely acceptable to the scientific community but, since it was preceded by Lord Rothschild's report, readers of the Green Paper were first confronted by his more dogmatic and less well-argued revolutionary changes. As a result many scientists and clinicians—including the author—reacted (perhaps over-reacted) vociferously. In the days before Christmas 1971, members of the Faculty of Medicine in my own University hurriedly arranged debates; by Christmas Eve a letter of protest to *The Times* had been prepared over a vast array of signatories. It was considered that scientific discovery is an activity of scientists and that additions to fundamental knowledge frequently proved, on application, to be of remarkable benefit to society. I am in no doubt that the vehemence of this reaction was due in large measure to the mode of Rothschild's presentation of his proposals. Not surprisingly public debate brought out the point that the massive investment by government in research now necessitated the forging of well-defined links between government and science with clearer definition of responsibility and accountability.

In the event, Lord Rothschild's recommendations were in large measure accepted by the government and the White Paper (Cmnd 5046) was published in July 1972.

The last sentence of the last paragraph of the White Paper summarizes its theme, and reads 'The new framework provides a partnership within which science will have more influence on the Government's central policy making activities than before, and which (framework) will contribute more directly and more effectively to the task of making the best use of science and technology for the needs of the community as a whole'. The six months that had passed between the publication of the Green and White Papers had taken some of the heat out of the immediate reaction to the former. It was now evident that the message of Rothschild was not merely an attack on research but was, in the main, a challenge to the customer (in our context, the health departments) to clarify what research was required to foster and improve the National Health Service. The tasks facing the health departments (and I put this in the context of the SHHD) were the setting up of a customer structure to define and commission research and implement the results where appropriate; an examination of existing funding arrangements; the establishment of an appropriate new relationship with the DHSS and the MRC; and, fundamental to all these, the appointment of a Scottish Home and Health Department Chief Scientist advised by a Chief Scientist Committee and supported by a Chief Scientist Organization.

3

The establishment of the Chief Scientist Organization within the Scottish Home and Health Department

The way in which the DHSS established the structure designed to implement the injunctions of the White Paper has been described by Cohen (3). Opportunity is taken here to outline the evolution of the Chief Scientist Organization in Scotland.

The Green Paper of November 1971 gave a clear indication of forthcoming events and so, without waiting for the advent of the subsequent White Paper, the Scottish Home and Health Department sought the advice of its Advisory Committee on Medical Research—a prestigious committee of academics set up following the establishment of the NHS in 1948 to scrutinize and advise on applications from the scientific community in Scotland for financial support through the Scottish Hospital Endowments Research Trust or from Secretary of State funds. Accordingly, the ACMR convened a conference at the University of Strathclyde in February of 1972 and invited representatives from the Scottish universities, the Medical Research Council, the DHSS, and the Nuffield Provincial Hospitals Trust. Discussion centred around the promotion, organization, and support of medical and dental research in Scotland in the light of the Green Paper. Several important principles were established which were later taken into account by the Department when acting upon the commands of the White Paper.

First, it was considered that in terms of its medical research potential it was inappropriate to consider Scotland as being equivalent to a large English region (as it was in population terms); it was different in several ways, notably by having four university medical schools which were favourable to the promotion and conduct of medical research, and it was suggested that it was important to think in terms of developing a research policy specifically for Scotland while, at the same time, collaborating fully at UK level.

Secondly, there was favourable comment on the existing relationships, at a personal level, between members of the ACMR and the professional staff of the SHHD and much stress was placed on the importance of maintaining, and strengthening, this relationship if the ACMR was to be replaced by a new research organization.

Thirdly, the meeting was in favour of the appointment of a Chief Scientist who would continue to practise clinically within the NHS (and so the appointment would be a part-time one), and who had gained some experience of the work of the MRC, the ACMR, and of the health departments.

Fourthly, recognizing that the ACMR had played a relatively passive role in as much as its activities had been almost exclusively related to making recommendations on the scientific merit of spontaneous applications for research grants, it was recommended that it, or its successor, must now accept a policy role. In order to do this effectively information would be required concerning the nature and amount of current research being done, the facilities available for research, and the fields in which research was considered to be most needed. To obtain this information there would require to be close liaison between the new research organization and such bodies as the universities, the SHHD, the Scottish Health Services Planning Council (once established), and the MRC in its role as the principal government agency for the promotion of medical research throughout the United Kingdom. It would also be of value to commission *ad hoc* working groups to study problem areas and invite 'state of the art' reports on particular health problems from individual experts.

Following the advice of the ACMR Conference, the SHHD evidently considered that the Regius Professor of Surgery in the University of Glasgow had, to an adequate degree, the qualifications specified for the post of part-time Chief Scientist. He accepted this appointment on two conditions: there should be no personal remuneration; that the teaching and clinical responsibilities of the University Department of Surgery be maintained by an SHHD contribution to the University of Glasgow to enable a vacant lectureship post to be upgraded to one at senior lecturer level. This latter condition permitted the appointment of a highly respected senior colleague, acknowledged within the Medical School as an outstanding teacher and surgeon. My appointment was confirmed in February of 1973.

The next step was to establish the Chief Scientist Committee. Once again the advice of the ACMR Conference was taken into consideration and the membership was drawn largely from senior members of university departments. The specialties covered the fields of surgery, psychiatry, pharmacology and therapeutics, pathology, medical sociology, general practice, obstetrics and gynaecology, social medicine, nursing studies, biology, computing and medicine; other disciplines would be represented in turn with changing membership of the committee. Thus the policy was established of involving academics directly in the process of bringing a scientific influence to bear on health service problems and, hopefully, on central policy-making activities. In an attempt to ensure this last important objective senior officers of the SHHD were also members of the Committee: the Chief Medical, Nursing, and Dental Officers, and the Chief Pharmacist. The ACMR had regularly had the benefit of the advice of the Secretary of the MRC (or his Deputy) and this fruitful association was continued by appointing the Second Secretary of the MRC to be a member of the CSC. It will be noted that the Chief Scientist Committee in Scotland had a continuing biomedical as well as a health service component. There were several reasons for this. First, it would ensure that the development of the Chief Scientist role in the SHHD would have an embracing influence on research in medicine and would provide an individual Scottish identity. Secondly, it would help to ensure a continuing good relationship with the Trustees of the Scottish Hospital Endowments Research Trust. Thirdly, it would permit an intellectual and educational dialogue among basic scientists, clinical scientists, and social scientists. Finally, it fulfilled a philosophy expressed at the February 1972 Conference that knowledge and experience should flow with equal freedom from practice to research and from research to practice; the research organization should be able to take account of the full range of scientific activities relevant to medical research and to improvement of the Health Service.

Simultaneously, the Chief Scientist office staff was being appointed under the leadership of a principal medical officer (PMO) with expertise in research management. Attendance of CSO staff at meetings of the Chief Scientist Committee ensured that scientific expertise, departmental views, and research management capability are all represented. It therefore constitutes a forum at which departmental views on needs, together with research views on design and feasibility can be debated.

A relatively simple research organization was evolving but it was evident that this would be of little avail unless the scientific community and the caring professions in Scotland could be actively involved at an early stage. It was decided, therefore, to hold a residential conference for invited representatives from the relevant bodies in order to give them an opportunity to contribute at the developmental stages. The Conference was held in the University of St Andrews in September 1973. After a preliminary general discussion, during which the conference gave full approval to the initial steps taken in setting up the Chief Scientist Organization, the membership met in syndicates to consider a number of particular issues. An attempt is made here to summarize the more important points raised.

It was agreed that in addition to full collaboration at UK level there should be an active research policy for Scotland, in the fields of both health services and biomedical research, and that it was a task for the CSC and CSO to formulate and execute the policy. It would clearly be essential to relate research endeavour to recognized health needs of the population, and in order to gain the information required to do this it would be necessary for the CSO to establish good communication throughout the NHS as well as with researchers in Scotland. In the beginning, without embarking on the traumatic exercise of endeavouring to arrange priorities, it would be a relatively simple matter to identify major health problems in Scotland such as alcoholism, ischaemic heart disease, perinatal mortality, etc. Again it was suggested that some areas within Scotland—away from teaching centres—could provide stable patient populations which could be fruitful bases for epidemiological research in relation to the natural history of a disease or to the roles of different categories of health services staff.

The need for an intensive scrutiny of nursing and nursing research was advocated. There was inadequate knowledge about the way in which staff were selected to fill the various nursing roles; training too, required assessment. It was accordingly suggested that consideration be given to the appointment of an *ad hoc* nursing research group to advise the CSC.

It was accepted that, before research funding of a project or programme was due to end, steps should be taken to see that adequate assessment was made. Particular attention would require to be given timeously to the possible development of a service commitment arising from the work.

The Department, as the customer, would not normally invite open tenders for a given commission but would negotiate a contract with the research director and team selected by the CSO as most appropriate to undertake the work; personal knowledge of research workers was a benefit of Scotland's being a small country.

The importance of the dissemination from the CSO of research results, and the need to feed the fruits of research back into the Health Service, was stressed. Commencing in the September 1974 issue of the *Health Bulletin* a section has regularly appeared under the heading 'The Chief Scientist Reports'.

The medical secretariat of the Advisory Committee on Medical Research had succeeded in establishing and maintaining rapport with research workers in the field and, while it was recognized that the responsibilities of the CSO officers had a much wider range than those of their predecessors, it was hoped that everything would be done to retain this form of personal contact. This would be of particular importance in underdeveloped disciplines or where research and training needed encouragement. It was recognized that some applications for research funding which failed the scrutiny of a scientific advisory committee might contain the germ of a good idea and feedback on such applications should be encouraged.

Finally, it was suggested that the growth and status of health services research would be advanced if an applicant's experience in this type of work was recognized as an important asset in making appointments to senior medical and nursing posts. It was further proposed that opportunity should be sought to include such experience in existing undergraduate medical and higher professional training courses.

The Chief Medical Officer, Sir John Brotherston, summed up the Conference. He emphasized that the CSO must first and foremost seek to improve the NHS in Scotland so that it might provide a better service and improve the health of the community. He considered that the coincidental major changes in NHS organization were fortunate in that there was now an explicit responsibility on the Department and on health boards to set their objectives and establish their priorities in a systematic fashion. He added that the initial requirement was information on health needs and that it would be for the CSC to identify situations where the basic knowledge required to meet a specific need was lacking and to encourage, and on occasions commission, the relevant research. He emphasized the need for the Department and the Health Service to be prepared to adopt an experimental and innovative approach to the delivery of health services, inviting persons with other types of skills to come and assist in the health services research process. He emphasized that it would be necessary to provide career opportunities in health services research and to establish long-term support for certain areas of the subject, for example, to discover what was the consumer's attitude and also to experiment in the delivery of medical care by alternative models. This latter example is an indication of how the CSO impinges on health service planning responsibility. There was a great need for communication and feedback to and from all concerned.

Robert Townsend (4), former Chairman of the Avis Rent-a-Car Corporation has given much sage advice to everyone who is or might be trapped in the sludge of 'organization-think'. Thus, 'before you commit yourself to a new effort, it is worth asking yourself a couple of questions: are we really trying to do something worthwhile, or are we just building another monument to some diseased ego? A decision to locate your new factory in Orlando or Yakima shouldn't be made hastily, nor without plenty of inputs from operating people and specialists.' The decision to hold the St Andrews Conference satisfied the last piece of advice, and the discussions and outcome indicated that the forthcoming exercise, though difficult, was worthwhile and had a real chance of at least modest success. The discussions had also clarified the broad responsibilities which would fall upon the CSO and these are now summarized. The CSO is responsible for advice to the Secretary of State on: (*a*) the scientific implications of objectives proposed for the Health Service in Scotland, and the scientific aspects of these objectives; (*b*) the promotion of an R & D plan to improve the provision and operation of particular health services; (*c*) the scientific assessment of specific research programmes and projects; (*d*) the maintenance of balanced support among the different fields of research. It would also be important to try to ensure the co-ordination of CSO activities with those of the corresponding organization within the DHSS and with those of the MRC. Finally, the CSO must give leadership and assistance to the NHS in a scanning process for new developments in the provision of health services, and encourage their experimental promotion when and where considered appropriate; the linking of medical research to health service sobjectives would clearly have the consequence that part of the R & D portfolio must be initiated by the Chief Scientist Organization.

The next step in establishing the full Chief Scientist Organization was to determine the structure considered to be necessary to fulfil its responsibilities and objectives. In doing so a simple principle was observed, namely, that the fewer committees the better, the membership be kept to the minimum compatible with the provision of adequate expertise, and that the number of meetings held should be few and related to the workload.

Similarly, in forming the Chief Scientist Office, no attempt was made to take advantage of the 'honeymoon period' by requesting a large professional and administrative secretariat and so it was decided to work on the principle that staffing should be related to developing workload—in keeping with the humorously expressed advice of Robert Townsend (4)!

All you have to do is look around you to see that modern organisations are only getting people to use about 20%—the lower fifth—of their capacities.

And the painful part is that God didn't design the human animal to function at 20%. At that pace it develops enough malfunctions to cause a permanent shortage of psychoanalysts and hospital beds.

THE CHIEF SCIENTIST OFFICE

Believing that close collaboration between professional (medical) and administrative officers of SHHD would be of vital importance in this new exercise, the secretariat comprises these two elements. A professional group is headed by a principal medical officer (PMO), and the administrative element by an assistant secretary (AS) who has departmental responsibilities in addition to his commitment to CSO. This close association between the two elements is again maintained between the Chief Scientist and the Under-Secretary as circumstances require; both elements are fused at the level of Secretary of the Department. Working relationships have been good and, in my view, the conduct of our work has been efficient.

The strength of the professional staff at this time, in addition to the PMO, is one SMO (full-time), three SMOs (each part-time), one nursing officer (part-time), one senior principal scientific officer (SPSO—part-time), and one senior scientific officer (SSO—full-time).

The administrative section of the secretariat, in addition to the principal (AS—part-time), consists of one senior executive officer, two higher executive officers, two executive officers, two clerical officers, and two clerical assistants.

The tasks of the CSO are many and varied, and the more important only will be described. First, in addition to servicing the Chief Scientist's Committee there is a need to service the four standing advisory committees which are subtended to the CSC, which provides over-all policy guidance. Secondly, the professional secretaries of these committees receive and process research applications which will be scrutinized by the relevant committees and, thereafter, be responsible for the research management of funded projects and programmes. Success in this area calls for good contact with research workers and the willingness to allocate sufficient time to receive, assimilate, and assess ideas from many sources. Advice to researchers should always be forthcoming and helpful and so it follows that the amount of advisory time spent with applicants and grant-holders is one of judgement, but I am convinced that this image of approachability must be maintained; as research agencies become larger they run the great risk of becoming unapproachable, mechanistic, and of losing the goodwill of the scientific community. Thirdly, the professional officers must maintain easy communication with the departmental administrative staff who have a depth of experience of service problems and service needs; during the past three years I have observed and appreciated the ease with which rapid exchanges of this sort can be made, and this in turn has led to a growing mutual respect and understanding. Fourthly, the Office plays a major role with the Department and the CSO Committees in identifying NHS problems and in establishing research priorities. Fifthly, liaison activities with the MRC and with the DHSS place a considerable burden on the professional staff because of the time required to scrutinize all relevant papers and because of the frequent need to attend meetings in London. The greater part of this effort is concerned with the handling of the health departments' commissioning funds for biomedical research: despite the importance of this responsibility, time spent in this way is lost to the forwarding of our prime objective of promoting research aimed at improving the health service in Scotland. The difficulties and problems encountered in endeavouring to implement the customer/contractor principle make it abundantly clear that this was one of the less inspired recommendations of Rothschild, certainly as applied to research in medicine.

The fact that some of the medical officers work on a part-time basis to the CSO may seem to accord poorly with the demands of the above workload, but it was considered important that CSO staff should not run the risk of becoming professionally isolated and, furthermore, work in two areas could be important for the career prospects of the officers concerned. It was also decided, in relation to the status and acceptance of the professional staff by the scientific community, that approval would be given to their seeking honorary appointments (limited to one or two sessions) in relevant academic departments. These decisions will hopefully ensure that research management, administration, and the scientific community have every opportunity to work in harness.

The Chief Scientist Committee. This committee's role has now evolved to an extent when its functions are now reasonably clear. First, it is responsible for the consideration, possible amendment, and approval of recommendations for policy developments proposed by its four specialized committees. Secondly, in the light of evolving policy and a review of the research portfolio in relation to this, it must determine annually the proportion of the CSO budget to be allocated to each committee. Thirdly, it will assist in the formulation of advice on R & D in the NHS in Scotland for the Scottish Health Services Planning Council, both directly and in response to requests for advice. Fourthly, it assists in the formulation of advice on biomedical research needs and priorities, particularly in relation to the use of commissioning funds to be allocated to the MRC; this has been done in close collaboration with the DHSS. I have already made reference to problems arising in the fulfilment of this responsibility and these are discussed in Chapter 4. Finally, it is the responsibility of this committee to identify and examine (directly, by setting up *ad hoc* expert groups, or by reference to one of its specialized committees) those areas within the Health Service where research might be expected to effect an improvement in the service or a reduction in the cost of its provision.

The membership of this committee has been planned to ensure that there is a nexus between the CSO and the policymaking elements in the health department. Thus, while the membership is largely made up of academics offering a variety of expertise, the chief officers of the department are also members. This arrangement was made as a step towards accepting one of the main challenges of the White Paper, namely, to ensure a partnership within which science would have a growing influence on central policymaking activities than before. Issues arise when judgement cannot be made purely on scientific grounds and political influences must be taken into consideration; in situations of this sort departmental input is of crucial importance.

A two-way flow of information between the CSC and its specialized committees is assured by the chairmen of these committees having membership of the CSC *ex-officio*.

The Biomedical Research Committee. This is the successor to the Advisory Committee on Medical Research. Of long and prestigious standing, the ACMR had been serviced at a high level and the scientific standards which it set were such that research workers in Scotland regarded the award of a grant from this committee as being the equivalent of one from the MRC. It functioned on the basis that awards should be made almost entirely on the criterion of scientific excellence; beyond this, little or no attempt was made to evolve a policy. Again, the ACMR advised the Scottish Hospital Endowments Research Trust on biomedical applications submitted separately to that body—a responsibility which the Biomedical Research Committee will continue to discharge. The MRC is the UK agency for biomedical research and the BRC will not be merely another source of biomedical research funds available to Scottish workers. The Second Secretary of the MRC is a member of the BRC and his advice and breadth of experience have been invaluable. The Committee is working towards the development of a policy for supporting biomedical research of an increasingly applied nature relevant to the objectives of the CSO and the particular health problems in Scotland. Criteria of significance in determining scientific policy have been agreed and are in operation. Management criteria which should help to decide relative priorities within a scientific policy have also been established (Appendix).

Health Services Research Committee. This is a key committee for the attainment of CSO objectives. In its initial work the committee faced the dilemma of endeavouring to balance the need to develop a health services research capability in Scotland against awarding support only to work of high scientific quality. The dilemma is a very real one. If the image and stature of this relatively new form of medical research is to improve to the point of acceptability by clinical and biological scientists, good standards must be set; on the other hand, until active academic departments pursuing health services research are available in sufficient number to produce a growing cadre of research workers progress may best be made by supporting work of adequate (rather than superlative) quality. Another temporary difficulty had to be overcome.

In contrast to traditional research committees where scientists from differing biological disciplines had become accustomed to working together, it was a new experience for social scientists, economists, clinicians, community physicians, nurses, etc., to work in harness and so there was an initial tendency for each to emphasize the contribution of his own particular discipline. However, even in the short space of three years, common objectives are increasingly appreciated, and initial successes are oiling the wheels of collaboration.

Recognizing that it would not be possible to evolve policy in a short time across the entire span of the committee's interests, and that it would also take time to determine an order of priorities, the decision was taken (with the approval of CSC) to examine research needs in a few areas which were clearly of great importance. Initially, working groups were set up to examine research needs in the health care of the elderly and for family planning; as a result active steps have been taken to implement some of the recommendations within a phased programme. Subsequently, other major problems have been identified to which the committee has given priority consideration; in each instance an *ad hoc* working group has been established, some have now reported, and feasible research is in progress or has been planned. It has been a matter of policy *not* to set up standing committees in priority fields, but instead to gain the in-depth advice of experts in the course of a short period of intense activity. In this way the tendency of our times to increase the number of permanent committees has been avoided.

Computer Research Committee. This committee was able to draw on the experience gained by its forerunner, the Research Committee of SACHHS. Concerned initially with 'peer group' assessment of spontaneous applications for support from the scientific community, the committee has now given considerable attention to policy development. It was encouraged to do so because of the high capital expenditure in this field, the problems of staff recruitment and career prospects, the limited number of centres capable of carrying out research of real significance to the NHS in Scotland, and the setting up of computer consortia in the

NHS. The importance of endeavouring to ensure that successful R & D would be implemented into service use was soon recognized and, with this important objective in view the committee, from an early stage, decided to meet in each Scottish University in turn, study the work in progress at first hand, and establish good communication with the senior administrators of the relevant area health board.

Recently it has become clear that the nature of the CRC's work has changed in so far as most applications for funding are concerned with the use of computers as a tool in medical research rather than to the performance of research into medical computing itself. If this trend continues, the time may come when it would be appropriate to disband this committee and refer grant applications involving computing techniques to BRC or HSRC. A reduction in the number of standing committees is a desirable aim, and every such committee must justify its establishment and its continued existence.

Equipment Research Committee. This was the last of the CSO specialized committees to be established. At an early stage it became clear that policy development would be a matter of considerable difficulty, particularly since its remit included the evaluation of commercially developed equipment. Appraised of the difficulties ahead, the CSO's equipment role was put under intense scrutiny, first by the CSO and subsequently with the assistance and advice of appropriate officers within the SHHD. The fundamental issues have now been clarified and, among the recommendations made, it has been decided to abolish this committee. There will be a new organization within the SHHD to replace the ERC consisting of an advisory group of the Planning Council with three sub-groups; one for equipment R & D; one for equipment evaluation; and one for prosthetics and orthotics. Because of the CSO's continuing interest in research aspects of equipment it has been agreed that the chairman of the advisory group will report to the Chief Scientist Committee.

The final meeting of the ERC will have taken place before this manuscript is in the hands of the printers.

In the past decade there has been a growing interest in problems of health care delivery and a rising appreciation of the need to study these problems in a scientific manner. Considerable impetus has been given to this movement by the injunction in the White Paper that Chief Scientist Organizations be established in relation to the health departments. The way in which the CSO in Scotland has been established has been described; time and continuous monitoring should indicate the success or failure of the operation. At this early stage the organization would seem to have some merits. The structure is simple, and already the small number of initially formed standing committees is being reduced. The essential lines of communication linking the organization with the scientific community and with the Department show few signs of obstruction and information is flowing satisfactorily—certainly as far as the CSO's activities within Scotland are concerned. I believe the decision to involve all participants in this important exercise from the outset to have been correct; I have little doubt that the imposition of a new organization without this consultation would have been regarded as another step towards growing bureaucracy and would have militated against progress. Although health service research is being encouraged and promoted particularly, the unity of research in medicine is recognized by the inclusion of biomedical and clinical research in CSO responsibilities; the desirability, in the longer term, of achieving a fine balance across the entire spectrum of medical research is recognized. In due course there will doubtless be a demand for information on the 'value' of research funded or commissioned by the CSO but even now I suspect that this will be exceedingly difficult, if not impossible, to provide. Cost/benefit criteria can be applied to the minority of research work, and here mainly in well-defined operational research studies. Can we cost advances in knowledge? I believe that it would be dangerous to make cost/benefit our principal criterion, for the reason that it is not only unrealistic but could lead to a restriction on the support of important research in the future. However, the CSO must ensure that it is able to demonstrate that its research portfolio is of high scientific quality, relevant to the improvement of the Health Service, and balanced so that it takes account of NHS problems and policies on the one hand and scientific feasibility, opportunity, and the availability of facilities on the other. Hopefully, it would also be in the position to show that research was being managed efficiently and that its advisory machinery was responsive to demands made upon it.

THE CHIEF SCIENTIST TO A HEALTH DEPARTMENT

Three appointments have so far been made to the post of Chief Scientist to a health department. Dr R. H. L. Cohen was appointed Chief Scientist to the DHSS in October 1972 and, very shortly thereafter, it was announced that Sir Douglas Black would succeed to this post in April 1973. I was appointed Chief Scientist to the SHHD in February 1973. I have just heard of the announcement, which brought me the greatest personal pleasure, of the election of Sir Douglas to the prestigious position of President of the Royal College of Physicians; my immediate reaction of pleasure registered, I began to ponder possible successors as Chief Scientist to the DHSS and this led me to consider the experience and qualities desirable in a Chief Scientist to a health department. Well aware of the possibility of personal bias, I discussed this interesting topic with a close friend and colleague who possessed the insight and background necessary to give a balanced opinion. As the discussion proceeded I became aware of my own deficiencies but, nevertheless, decided to put on record from my experience of four years as a Chief Scientist the essential qualifications for the post. I would emphasize that I have not sought the view of my good friends Dr Cohen and Sir Douglas Black. Recognizing the vulnerable position in which I place myself, I now offer personal views.

First, I am in no doubt that it is essential that a Chief Scientist should have a strong background of research experience, both by involvement at the bench and as a scrutineer of applications for research support. Secondly, as he will be involved to a large extent in research directed towards the health services I believe that he should be a medical graduate and, preferably, one who has spent much of his life in close association with patient care. Thirdly, experience of administration and of the Civil Service are relatively unimportant provided the Chief Scientist has (as it has been my good fortune to have) the support of high-quality staff in the Chief Scientist Office, particularly in the area of research management. Fourthly, an understanding of the role and functioning of the Medical Research Council, preferably by previous involvement, would be advantageous; the development of a meaningful policy for the health sciences demands close collaboration between the MRC and the health departments, based on mutual trust and understanding. Fifthly, the man appointed to the post of Chief Scientist should come from outwith the health department and, as it will take him some time to comprehend the system, he should be appointed for a period of at least five years; the CSO staff can do much but it is the job of the Chief Scientist to influence the direction of affairs and he is unlikely to be able to do this by an appointment of shorter tenure. Sixthly, those responsible for appointing a Chief Scientist should try to find an individual acceptable to the Civil Service who, at the same time, commands the respect of the scientific community. Should the Chief Scientist hold the appointment on a whole-time or on a part-time basis? I find this a very difficult question and the answer must, to some extent, depend on the scale of his activities. There can be no doubt that these are much less in relation to the SHHD than to the DHSS; for myself, I have found considerable advantage to be Chief Scientist while retaining real involvement in clinical work, close contact with fellow clinicians, and opportunity for regular discussions with research workers. For operations on a larger scale there could be merit in following the example of the Royal College of Physicians and Surgeons of Glasgow whereby the President spends the two previous years as Visitor (Vice-President) acquiring the experience essential for his promotion (assured) to Presidency; he is thus prepared to grasp the opportunity to exert his influence on the course of affairs. There could be merit in appointing a Chief Scientist and a Deputy Chief Scientist, each for a period of two or three years; so that in this way continuity would be maintained and both men would run little risk of losing viable contact with their parent departments (for example a university clinical department). There are several variations on this theme.

within the Scottish Home and Health Department

It will be of more than passing interest to me personally, especially in the light of the above postulations, to meet the successor to Sir Douglas Black.

APPENDIX

Biomedical Research Committee

A. CRITERIA DETERMINING SCIENTIFIC POLICY SIGNIFICANCE (IN ORDER OF IMPORTANCE)

1. *Health service importance*

Research which may lead to greater effectiveness of the National Health Service in Scotland, or to greater efficiency by improving organization or functioning with a consequent freeing of resources.

2. *Excellence of study field*

Research of intrinsically high scientific value.

3. *Excellence of research workers, or scientific opportunity*

Research to be undertaken by exceptionally high-quality individuals or teams, or because an excellent scientific opportunity is otherwise available.

4. *Pervasiveness of the activity*

Research (*a*) likely to lead to advances in other fields as well as the primary care field, or (*b*) which can be implemented on a wide front.

5. *Significance for training of scientific manpower*

Research which will include the training or re-training of research workers, particularly in a field where they are few.

B. MANAGEMENT CRITERIA WHICH MAY HELP TO DETERMINE RELATIVE PRIORITIES WITHIN A SCIENTIFIC POLICY

(*a*) *Dependence on departmental support*

Research unlikely to be supported otherwise.

(*b*) *Timing*

Research which should start or be stepped up within up to three years if the expected benefits are to be obtained.

(*c*) *Availability of scientific manpower*

Research proposed because a suitable research worker or team is available.

4

The commissioning of biomedical research

In the White Paper of July 1972 the Government finally endorsed the customer/contractor principle, together with an accompanying transfer to executive departments of a proportion of research council funds (25 per cent in the case of the MRC). Conditions were not placed on the use of this transferred money but the expectation was that it would be used to commission research from the MRC dependent on the needs of the health departments. The latter therefore became the customers and had to be accountable for the sums paid to the MRC as contractors and, in so doing, had to be satisfied that the programmes of work equated with the total payment.

Prior to my appointment as Chief Scientist to the SHHD it had been proposed that the *Panel on Medical Research* (serviced by the DHSS but working jointly with Scotland and Wales) would be established to be responsible for advising on commissioned biomedical research, including the use of funds transferred from the science vote of the Department of Education and Science. It seemed to me that the members of this large committee would find it very difficult to understand the rules of this totally new game and I was strongly in favour of beginning on a smaller scale, suggesting that the responsibility should in the beginning centre around the two Chief Scientists supported by the chief medical officers of the health departments (or their deputies). In the event the organization established to deal with the deployment of 'transferred' or commissioning funds was the Panel on Medical Research. Major difficulties were experienced in practice. The Panel lived dangerously! In essence, it was being asked to advise on the relevance of MRC-supported work to health department needs without being provided with information either about those needs or about the total UK and international research efforts in the various fields. Skirmishes with this impossible task led to growing frustration. Again, in the development of research policies the difficulties of the MRC Boards and the health departments (at the PMR) in considering the same issues from different standpoints separately at different fora were highlighted very clearly. I am in no doubt that this could have been a much more realistic and productive exercise if it had been conducted in one place by a small group rather than through two different yet similar thinking biomedical advisory groups with overlapping membership.

Again, the Panel adopted unrealistic views on the amount of influence it could expect to assert on the commissioning programme in the short term and, in consequence, felt even further frustrated. This was because the commissioning programme was organized on the principle of 'broad commissions', that is, grouping of research projects and programmes under a theme heading; as various components of research terminated the idea was that new research relevant to the objectives of the particular commission would be slotted in. It was planned that the commissions would be reviewed every five years, so that one-fifth of the total programme (currently more than £10 million annually) would be reviewed each year. Thus the extent of possible change in any one year was limited and the room for manoeuvre was diminished further by the fact that almost all of existing MRC research was clearly of relevance to the health departments. It is here that the kernel of the difficulty lies: in the area of biomedical research the MRC has the experience and scientific personnel to function as an efficient contractor whereas, in contrast, the health departments cannot reasonably claim to have either.

It is fortunate that this complex exercise was not subjected to a cost/benefit study! There is no doubt that the mechanism established for dealing with the transferred funds was over-elaborate, involved an excess of work by the staff of the health departments (and in this regard I am deeply conscious of the particular demands made of my colleagues in the DHSS who accepted the responsibility of servicing the PMR and providing an officer to serve each of the new MRC Boards which, as a result of MRC reorganization, now include the Neurosciences Board, the Cell

Board, the Systems Board, the Tropical Medicine Research Board, and the Environmental Medicine Committee—in addition to the Council itself) and far too much valuable time from members of the scientific community. From my own viewpoint, I was concerned that these arrangements involved a very considerable proportion of the time of my own CSO professional staff in preparing input material for the PMR and in scrutinizing all research applications to MRC boards. My concern lay not only in the fact that I considered the work to be lacking productivity but that, in responding to the heavy demands of this complex system set up to secure the undertaking of relevant biomedical research by the MRC, we would be deflected from our main purpose of organizing health services research.

A series of discussions at officer level involving both Chief Scientists and members of the PMR failed to resolve the serious difficulties which had arisen in practice, and the view that this committee structure required revision was confirmed by a review of the DHSS/CSO organization commissioned by the Department and undertaken by Professor Kogan of Brunel University. It is perhaps unfortunate that Kogan concentrated on existing mechanisms and their shortcomings, rather than taking a detached overview of the tasks and how they might best be undertaken.

Reviewing the situation at this stage it should have been abundantly clear that the central problem facing the health departments was the difficulty of determining their biomedical research needs. With their strengthened research capacity through CSOs they had become better equipped to progress towards definition of their service problems and determine and design appropriate health service research; they were not equipped to determine biomedical research needs relevant to these problems; this expertise rests with the MRC and to duplicate this machinery would be an act of folly. I have indicated earlier that the MRC was moving increasingly into the fields of applied research and epidemiology and that a continued evolution in this direction would have been preferable to the Rothschild recommendation that funds be suddenly transferred; while I think it unlikely that the need would have arisen, it would have been better if this possibility had been held as a threat for the future if the MRC had failed to continue to increase the momentum of its response to health department needs. However, we were faced with the problem and the need remained to have a 'Rothschild' relationship of some sort between the health departments and the MRC for biomedical research. There was therefore no alternative but to restructure the system and attempt to make its successor much less complex and as effective and efficient as possible.

Following a series of informal discussions between those involved, culminating in an official meeting between the two Chief Scientists and senior officers of both departments, it was proposed that the PMR be replaced by a new joint Chief Scientists' Group. The proposals for the role, membership, and working of this new group were accepted by the MRC and by the health departments. In contrast to the PMR the group was numerically small consisting of the Chief Scientists and chief medical officers (or deputies) of the DHSS and SHHD, a senior professional research management officer from each department, a research management administrator from the DHSS (an officer of equivalent rank from the SHHD would attend as required), a nominee from the MRC and one from the Welsh Office. The Group is responsible for the supervision of all aspects of research management staff work in the commissioning of biomedical research from the MRC, it is executive, and co-ordinates and advises on any biomedical aspects of the work of the Research Liaison Groups (RLGs) in the DHSS and of the work of the Chief Scientist Committee in the SHHD. I believe that it would have been better to have started with this simple arrangement as it would have allowed for amendment and expansion in the light of experience. The underlying principle on which the Group will work is that the health departments should concentrate on defining problems and the MRC on defining biomedical research relevant to these problems. Whether this simplified arrangement would have been effective may never be known.

Growing financial stringency has resulted in severe staffing cuts throughout government departments including the health departments, and it is now realized that the staff work for even this simplified procedure is unlikely to be forthcoming. In the summer of 1976, after discussions with the DHSS Chief Scientist and senior officers, the then Minister of State, Dr David Owen, expressed concern at the detailed staff intensive work required for the existing arrangements and made it very clear that he wished to see a shift in emphasis of the MRC's programme brought about by a statement of broad priorities. As a result the Chief Scientists and officers of the health departments have given detailed consideration to further simplifying and amending the arrangements for the control of health department biomedical research funds. The new approach is under discussion as I write but the underlying principles can be summarized. First the health departments' input to the development of biomedical research should take the form of an annual statement of health problems and priorities; these would be presented in broad outline initially but as the system developed it would be hoped that more detailed statements of health problems, resulting from a closer analysis of service questions, could be presented. The MRC, in response, would set out their proposals for the development of relevant biomedical research. Thereafter, annually, the MRC would present a report of progress made in implementing health department requirements and the departments would determine the level of financial support for the following financial year and give an indication for subsequent years. In addition to this broad approach it would be open to the health departments to place specific commissions for research up to an agreed financial maximum for each year. I regard it as very important that we aim for a very simple approach to the first year, on the understanding that formats can be adjusted in the light of experience for later years. I am optimistic that this approach will prove to be more effective and require much less effort; the fact that it has been in part forced upon us by financial cut-backs indicates that these may have their benefits. Townsend has words appropriate to this situation:

> A tight budget brings out the best creative instincts in man. Give him unlimited funds and he won't come up with the best way to a result. Man is a complicated animal. He only simplifies under pressure. Put him under some financial pressure and he will scream in anguish. Then he will come up with a plan which, to his own private amazement, is not only less expensive but also faster and better than his original proposal . . .

Fortunately, despite the intractability of the commissioning process, the relationships between the health departments and the MRC have been maintained and there is a continued desire to collaborate for the best interests of research in medicine and the health care of our people.

5

Health services research

It is futile to continue argument and debate on the relative importance of biomedical, clinical, and health services research. Sharp boundaries do not exist between them, and together they form the spectrum of health sciences. They are dependent on each other and all must be taken into consideration in the formulation of a research policy. It is in the interest of health scientists, and in the interest of the country as a whole, to promote and encourage research policies which will maintain an effective balance. It is, however, helpful to use the traditional classification as an introduction to the development and growth of research directed towards the solution of health service problems.

Biomedical research is hallowed by tradition and is referred to by some, quite erroneously, as 'pure' research. I do not regard research as being either pure or impure, but I subscribe to an important difference between good research and bad research and these are adjectives which may be applied to any form of scientific activity. Biomedical research deals with the causation and mechanisms of disease and so the product is an increase in fundamental knowledge some or all of which can be applied to human needs when the time is opportune. There are real dangers at this time of financial stringency and national insecurity that fundamental research may be given a low priority. If research on immediate problems is favoured to the extent of ignoring long-term needs a state of imbalance would occur which could take many years to correct.

Clinical research, which deals with the clinical aspects of disease, diagnosis, and treatment, developed effectively in the second quarter of this century. Initially regarded by basic scientists as something less than 'pure' it has acquired respectability largely due to the growth of clinical academic departments in response to the Flexner Report. When the MRC established its twin board structure, the Biological Research Board was complemented by a Clinical Research Board.

During the past half century a growing collaboration has slowly but importantly developed between biologists and clinical scientists which has resulted in significant advances in our understanding of many diseases and in our capacity to treat afflicted patients.

Health services research, a relative newcomer to the triad of health sciences, has developed over the last decade in response to growing problems in our centrally funded public health service. It is perhaps too early for it to have infiltrated the service to the extent that it influences attitudes and ambitions but it is imperative that it will eventually do so. In a period of steady financial growth it was not appreciated that an unlimited service could ever fail to be provided; Wildavasky's 'Law of Medical Money' was fulfilled and health care costs rose to equal the available amount of money (5). Resources are now limited in this time of economic stringency and doctors and scientists must play their part in working out solutions and policies directed towards the best use of these resources.

The health departments and the recently established Chief Scientist organizations were faced, in addition to the impact of economic pressures, with consequences which arose to some extent from the way in which the National Health Service had developed. Policies had been limited to relatively few areas; a firm base for the quantification and assessment of the relative importance of perceived problems within the NHS was lacking; priorities for resource allocation were either undefined or ill-defined; until a few years before the White Paper there had been under-investment in research directed towards an improvement in the NHS; research proposals had arisen in an unsolicited way and so the research portfolios were of varying quality and lacked focus; experience was inadequate for the definition of research which could contribute to a solution of problems in the commissioning of such research, and in research management.

In describing the establishment and structure of the CSO (Scotland) I emphasized that an important feature is that scientific expertise, departmental views, and research management expertise (CSO Office) are all represented in committee membership, thus constituting a forum at which departmental views on needs and research on feasibility and design can be freely debated. Has there been recognizable progress?

The CSO was established prior to the Scottish Health Services Planning Council and so, in the first instance, it had to determine its own research policies and priorities. The various working groups at the St Andrews Conference separately produced a checklist of NHS problems meriting study; the total checklist amounted to more than forty items! The phrase 'get your priorities right' rolls off the tongue in all walks of life today, but if this is to be taken seriously it requires both time and effort which could delay action on initiating research to solve even a few problems. As a first step, CSC commissioned a paper from the Information Services Division on 'Health Problems in Scotland'. No serious attempt was made to establish precise priorities (without study in depth, this would not have been possible), but several problems were identified as being major ones and of especial relevance to health in Scotland. Secondly, at each of its quarterly meetings the CSC invited an expert to review his own field in depth and associated with these presentations there was usually an accompanying paper by the ISD attempting to set forth the relevant disease burden to the health service. Thirdly, the HSRC invited administrative and medical department staff to attend their meetings with the specific purpose of presenting identified problems. These steps taken and bearing in mind that an NHS problem or priority area is not necessarily a research priority (which will depend on such factors as resources, feasibility, appropriate research workers, etc.) *ad hoc* working groups were established in a few selected areas and required to report back expeditiously to the CSC or the HSRC. Where the identification of a problem had been confirmed and research towards its solution regarded as feasible, the next step in the commissioning procedure was to encourage applications for support from the most appropriate source of relevant expertise. This has usually resulted in a formal application to be assessed on its merits by the HSRC or/and the CSC and a decision reached as to acceptability, modification, or rejection of the proposal. On this basis work has been commissioned on family planning, geriatrics, selected problems of alcohol, 'strokes', management of head injuries (resulting from a specialist review presentation to the CSC), health economics (resulting from departmental/HSRC discussions), and dental research.

The first stage of the commissioning process—the identification of a researchable problem—is as described above. The second stage of the process, which is to encourage applications to meet the research needs, has been approached in several ways and early experience has shown that this flexible approach should continue to be pursued. First, interest in a research field has been stimulated by publishing the recommendations of an *ad hoc* working group. Secondly, a working paper (incontinence) or a preliminary study (use of day hospitals) has been commissioned directly; consideration of these may lead to the encouragement of a formal application for funding of work on agreed facets of the problem. Thirdly, in relation to family planning, the working group was reconvened and given the remit to define the objectives, research methodology, and designs which, when endorsed by the HSRC and CSC, were used as a basis for negotiation with interested research workers. Fourthly, opportunity has been taken to exploit existing project activity in an accepted priority area, as was done in the decision to establish a health economics unit (University of Aberdeen/Grampian Area Health Board). Finally, one of the recommendations of the advisory group on dental research was that a 'dental research group' should be established within a Scottish academic dental department; accordingly, letters inviting competitive tenders for work to meet specific requirements have been sent to the appropriate universities. No matter the approach used to encourage applications, the final decision for each has been based on scientific scrutiny by the full membership of the appropriate committee.

No serious procedural difficulty has arisen with this flexible approach to the commissioning of health services research, but it is appreciated that conflict could arise between an expert working party and the main committee as a result of enforcement of the final requirement; unfavourable scrutiny at the final stage would destroy the efforts of the working party. For this reason, modifications of the procedure are being considered at the present time which would allow the HSRC to delegate responsibilities for negotiation, development, and recommendation of formal approval of commissioned research; the existing imposition of limits on expenditure will ensure that ultimate responsibility for making over-all financial recommendations would remain with the committee.

The future in health services research. Reviewing the progress to date it may be said that the CSO has taken the first few halting steps. It has established what hopefully will be an increasing dialogue between researchers and the SHHD and, in doing so, has demonstrated that this can help in defining specified problems in the health service. The problems defined, experience is gradually being gained in designing relevant research, how to commission this, and how to manage it. Each of the health service research units in Scotland has received a chief scientist visit following which the on-going programme of work was either approved or modified (Table 1); health service research expenditure for 1975/6 (Table 2) gives some indication of the span of research activities. Encouraging though this may be it is far too early to claim any real success for this relative newcomer to the family of health sciences. Although it uses the same science, evidence of a firm scientific discipline will be required before it gains an acceptable image. But I forecast that it will do so and that its growth will be along similar lines to that of clinical research so that, in due time, it will have equal acceptance by the scientific community. Of equal importance, the quality of the research work done will determine the strength of the link forged between the researchers

TABLE 1. *Health services research units*

Health Services Operational Research Unit, University of Strathclyde
Nursing Research Unit, University of Edinburgh
Scottish General Practitioner Research Support Unit, University of Dundee
Social Paediatric and Obstetric Unit, University of Glasgow
Hospital Health Services Research Unit, Western Infirmary, Glasgow*
Health Economics Research Unit, University of Aberdeen

* Funded jointly by the Nuffield Provincial Hospitals Trust and the Scottish Home and Health Department.

TABLE 2. *Health service research expenditure 1975/6*

Research area	*Expenditure (£000)*
Health service practice	75
Health service planning and management	59
General research support, training, and methodology	28
Nursing	48
General practice	11
Maternal and child health	35
Geriatric and mental health	27
Surgery and medicine	28
Others (dentistry, screening, occupational health)	11
All areas	322

and those responsible for providing the health service. The pattern and rate of change will depend on the easing of a variety of constraints.

First, implementation of results offers a formidable problem for the future but it is already clear that effective implementation will require the involvement of the service administrator in the research from its outset; he must approve the aims of the study, follow its progress, and be enthusiastic about implementation of a successful outcome of the research—even if the results make his life more difficult! The presentation of results on completion of research is most unlikely to be welcomed if changes in the service are demanded unexpectedly.

Secondly, it must be recognized that many of the health problems facing us today require contributions from a range of disciplines outwith the biological sciences: economics, statistics, epidemiology, ethics, and sociology. How can these contributions be ensured? Just as clinical research gained momentum from the multiplication of clinical academic units within universities and their growing collaboration with basic science departments, the growth and status of health services research will depend on the involvement of university departments of economy, sociology, etc., working in close collaboration with clinical scientists, doctors, and nurses. I am not unmindful of the tendency for scholars in a particular discipline to confine activities within the parent department, nor of the fact that universities are not organized in a way which encourages easy transgression of rigid departmental boundaries. A solution of this difficulty would be facilitated by the gradual introduction of these non-traditional disciplines into the undergraduate medical teaching programme. I anticipate outcries from those who regard curricula as already overcrowded to an extent which militates against the provision of a university education, and I find myself in near agreement with this view. I would argue, however, that it is not necessary for each discipline to have its rigid period of teaching time but rather that teachers in several disciplines participate together in specified teaching sessions. On one day each week my professional colleague in general practice joins me in teaching my surgical clinic: this arrangement prevents me from concentrating solely on the surgical aspects of a patient's problem to the exclusion of his personal anxieties and his family and social background; similarly, it is possible that my colleague gains a heightened understanding of the importance of appropriate early referral, diagnosis, and management. Teachers in one discipline have much to learn from their colleagues from other disciplines, and I believe that this process is facilitated when teachers are exposed together to the searching and critical questioning of young people. If health service problems are presented and considered in this manner the succeeding generation of doctors will acquire the right admixture of knowledge, skills, and reasoning from the relevant disciplines to be in a position to advance the prospects for high-quality health service research. If research is to permeate the service, enthusiasm must be engendered within our medical schools and given continuous nourishment throughout postgraduate training.

Thirdly, the need for health services research still lacks general acceptance—an attitude which is surely difficult to sustain at a time when stark issues confront the NHS. The purpose of research is to answer questions and solve problems. In the absence of problems related to the delivery of health care there is no need for health services research. But who would deny the existence of problems and that many do not fall within the ambit of biomedical and clinical research? While some of these are soluble and therefore merit research now, difficulties in methodology should not be underestimated. However similar problems faced, and continue to challenge, the clinical scientist who is frequently confronted with difficulties greater than those of his basic scientist colleague in planning well-controlled studies: his correct concern for the safety of patients under his care presents a difficulty which rarely confronts the molecular biologist. Herein lies part explanation of the former criticism that research, other than basic research, is 'soft' as opposed to 'hard'. Fortunately, the philosophy of the unity of the health sciences is gaining ground and the difficulties encountered by each are more generally recognized.

Fourthly, growing economic pressures are already leaving no alternative to the making of difficult choices, which means identification of priorities. We can no longer avoid taking into consideration the human and social costs of modern medicine, the quality of life and other ethical considerations. This can be brought into sharp focus by a consideration of the effects of advances in the management of renal failure and in the surgical treatment of coronary artery disease. In the first, patients with renal failure can be maintained by haemodialysis or be offered good-quality life by a successful kidney transplant: dialysis for all in need is exceedingly costly and the present public attitude to organ donation restricts surgical endeavours. In the second, evidence is growing that early surgical intervention by vein grafting will extend the expectation of life and improve the quality of life in middle-aged individuals with early disease of the coronary arteries. Should resources be preferentially given to this service as against the care of the elderly who have given, but can no longer give, of their efforts to national productivity? Planning of the health services to our people means choosing; as medicine advances, increasingly difficult choices will be encountered; the choices will involve ethical and moral considerations but decisions could be helped by the availability of reliable information from relevant health services research.

Fifthly, more attention will require to be given to the development of a career structure for research staff. Rapid growth in health services research in the past few years has made it difficult to determine the form which this should take but time is now of the essence. Additional constraints have arisen in the form of extra duty payments and inflexible training programmes. A solution will not be easy and this important matter is given separate consideration later.

Finally, doctors have been trained traditionally on the principle of personal responsibility for the care of the individual patient and I would not demur from this philosophy. However, we have no alternative but to think also in terms of groups of patients. We must ask ourselves the total problem of coronary artery disease in our society, consider the resources required for its best management, and assess the benefit to be expected. This attitude of inquiry, applicable to many disease states, will become mandatory for several reasons: the limitation of available resources; the increasing awareness of our patients about the availability of treatment and the related growing demand for equality of care. The answers to such questions cannot be plucked out of the air, but will depend on the outcome of well planned and continuing research endeavour. Far from conveniently going away, problems and choices of this sort will increase. Good health services research can help in choosing and so this moiety of research in medicine must be encouraged and high standards set for its development. In making this assertion I do not infer that there should be a reduction in biomedical or clinical research. Advances here will lead to a greater understanding of the causes of disease which in turn will lead to improvements in management and provide clues for prevention. The three branches of research in medicine overlap and it will be obvious that research in relation to prevention belongs to each group. Although the immediate product of each type of research differs, all share the same great objective—the conquest of ill health and an increased expectancy and quality of life.

The concept that biomedical research and health service research are complementary pursuits, and that careful monitoring is required to ensure the maintenance of a proper balance, has been emphasized by the US President's Science Advisory Committee's Panel on Health Services Research and Development (1972).

> The focus in health services R & D is on making biomedical knowledge available to treat, control and eliminate disease and to restore function or minimise disability, rather than on the development of that knowledge. Therefore biomedical research and health services research are complementary, although at times the boundaries between them are blurred. The success of the former

implies the need for the latter. If we fail to invest adequately in health services research to improve the availability of knowledge developed in the laboratory, we cannot realise the full benefits of our investment in biomedical research . . . Increased funding for health services research should not be undertaken at the expense of basic investigations into the causes and treatments of diseases. Without aggressive investment in biomedical research, health services have little to contribute. The budgets for biomedical and health services research have to be established independently on the basis of potential return per dollar, *by those with some understanding and vision.* At the same time, it should be recognised that access to the fruits of biomedical research depends in large measure upon the organisation and financing of effective and efficient health services . . . it is more reasonably argued that in view of the size of the health care 'crisis', the Federal government's stated objectives, and the public's expectations, we should increase the percentage of Federal funds invested in improving the efficiency, availability and quality of health services at this point in time. Let there be no misunderstanding, however, that this increased emphasis on health services R & D should be accompanied by reduced expenditures on biomedical research. Indeed, as health services are improved, the demand for usable biomedical knowledge will increase.

The Health Services Research Board. In the immediate post White Paper period much attention—perhaps too much—was given to the development of the structure of the new research organization and less to a clarification of how it would work and develop when put under stresses and strains. As one result of early discussions, the health departments and the MRC agreed to establish a Health Services Research Board (HSRB) on the lines of the MRC boards, including a budget and executive powers. It was to be lodged within, and serviced by, the DHSS on behalf of the health departments. Its main function was to advise on and provide support for programmes in health services research intended to lead to the better operation or improvement of the Health Services in the whole of Great Britain except for: biomedical research which is to be commissioned from the MRC; the specialized department R & D programmes related to computers, supply and equipment, and building for which specialized arrangements already existed. It should be noted that health service research projects (funded for up to three years) would be dealt with separately by the DHSS and SHHD, whereas programmes of research (long-term support or unit support) merited consideration at a UK level. On this basis the CSO (SHHD) agreed that the HSRB would assess Scottish programmes of health services research and assess the work of Scottish units in the field.

In the meantime the DHSS had begun to develop a system of Research Liaison Groups (RLGs). Each Group consisted of Policy Division and Research Management Division staff and independent scientists. The established RLGs had begun to formulate health service research policy, in some cases in a markedly effective way (Kogan Report). In consequence, the HSRB, before it had even begun to function, was left with virtually no role since it did not require to evaluate applications for funding nor could it contribute to policy development: a decision-making role lost, the most the Board could do was to act in an advisory capacity to the health departments and to the MRC. In consequence the initial agreement of the CSO (SHHD) to seek the Board's advice on proposed programmes of research, and to let it review ongoing programmes, was withdrawn with the agreement of the CSO (DHSS). As described earlier, programmes of research within Scotland are now agreed by the CSC in the light of recommendations made by the HSRC.

The HSRB met on a few occasions to deal with progressively diminishing agendas. It became clear that this was an unnecessary committee and it was disbanded by the mutual agreement of the health departments and the MRC.

In the future, the CSO (SHHD) will undoubtedly identify some areas of health services research which are relevant to the UK as a whole and in which they would wish to involve the DHSS as partner: health services research is mainly a matter for the health departments and no difficulty in continuing to coordinate our efforts in this field are envisaged.

Those of us involved in the establishment of the HSRB and of the PMR have no alternative but to concede that a basic rule was broken, namely, that no committee should be introduced without a very clear conception of its function and that this is capable of fulfilment.

6

Medical research and the universities

Medical research in this country has depended to a considerable extent on the contribution by universities to the nation's over-all scientific effort. The greater part of our non-industrial medical research is conducted in university departments and this holds for biological, clinical, and health services research. Again, increasing sophistication of research techniques and the need to involve the expertise of several disciplines in an attack on major health problems, means that research must frequently be undertaken in an environment where the necessary disciplines coexist: the universities alone fulfil this requirement. Finally, the universities have an important role in training scientists, thereby maintaining the nation's research capability. It would be true to say that the maintenance in this country of a university system that includes a sufficiency of scientific work, research, and training in the highest international class is essential for the continuance and development of the scientific work of the nation as a whole.

Firm in this belief, the Medical Research Council has operated the 'dual support system'. Public funds are made available in a non-selective manner through the University Grants Committee to provide a basic level of support for the research of university departments; at the same time a selective division of public funds is made through the research councils by the award of grants to support work of high scientific quality.

This system has worked well but in the last few years the economic situation in this country and the fight against inflation have, as in other national activities, led to severe cuts in the funds available for education and science. The universities have had to reconcile themselves to accepting an increase in the intake of undergraduate students in circumstances of acute financial stringency; teaching time has had to take precedence over research time and this change in emphasis has been exaggerated by the freezing of staff vacancies. The research councils have been endeavouring to adjust to the prospect of a no-growth situation for some years ahead. It is not surprising, therefore, that great strains have been placed on the dual-support system for research within universities. Even so, despite the fact that the research councils have the responsibility of maintaining their own establishments and external staff they have decided, as a matter of policy, to continue their support to universities and, as far as possible, ensure a parity between the support of research in universities on the one hand and their own establishments on the other.

Stresses are being created which show signs of causing unrest among medical scientists leading to a change in their attitudes and commitment. If government strives to control this worsening situation, as surely it should do, it will begin to feel the need for research and evaluation of the health care system to help in making and enforcing its decisions. Continuation of present constraints on university funding will steadily reduce the research base and it is to be hoped that the vital need to maintain this base is recognized before it is too late. The decline in support has rendered the climate for careers in research unattractive, there is a creeping erosion of the base for research in our universities, and action must be taken to ensure that the research environment is sustained and that a sufficiency of health research of merit will survive through the pressures of the next decade.

It is of interest that the Commission on Post-Secondary Education in Ontario has recently pointed out that there are dangers for both education and research in tying them too closely together. There may be a lesson for us here. In the past few years university funding has been related mainly to student numbers and teaching commitments and this to the gradual exclusion of research support. The time has come for consideration to be given to separate teaching and research funding to universities. The extent of funding for research should depend upon the location of the best research workers, and this will inevitably produce some differentiation of the university system throughout the country. There will be some with major strengths in many areas, some with strengths in limited areas and some with modest research but few major strengths. As Mustard (6) has pointed out, 'most societies regardless of their ideology have found some differentiation in the university system necessary as far as maintaining meritorious research and graduate programs is concerned'. Referring to Canada, he goes on:

> if this is brought into being it will be in our country's interests to encourage our able undergraduates and graduate students to study in the centres in this country that meet their needs. An adequate national scholarship program to encourage mobility of the students would be necessary. Surely there is an advantage to a country if it encourages its able youth to move around during their post-secondary education experiences. Some of these individuals will be future leaders in different sectors of our society. If enough of them have a national perspective they might help contribute to the forces that enable a country to maintain its national identity . . . members of the research community will have to make adjustments. These will include more public responsibility and accountability and an acceptance of the fact that all universities are not, and cannot be, equal in research.

Reference has been made to the dual-support system whereby the research councils supplement the basic research support given to universities through the University Grants Committee. There is also an increasing need for the health departments, committed as they are to encourage research directed towards the improvement of the Health Service, to consolidate a similar agreement with the universities and medical schools. Since all three organizations are concerned with medical education, research and, in general, the improvement of medical care the concept of a triple-support system merits exploration.

According to my information the UGC consults directly with the DHSS in the consideration of such problems as resource allocations to universities in England and Wales, whereas there is a less direct line of communication between the UGC and the SHHD. I suggest that Scotland is in some ways different from England as far as medical education and health are concerned. In population terms Scotland may be the equivalent of a large English region, but it should be remembered that it has eight universities, four with medical schools graduating over 20 per cent of the doctors in the United Kingdom. Again, the National Health Service was introduced in Scotland by a separate Health Act, as was the reorganization of the NHS in 1974. My concern is that decisions made in the context of the London and English provincial medical schools may be applied even if not relevant to the Scottish situation. Firmly opposed to a separate UGC for the Scottish universities, I advocate that there should be a Scottish Affairs Committee of the UGC, or some similar mechanism. A matter of immediate concern is the resource allocation to universities with medical schools and their related teaching hospitals. A formula has almost been agreed for England (SHIFT), but the variables taken into consideration in the development of this formula are not all relevant to the Scottish scene. The difficulty of the SHHD adopting a different line from the DHSS is recognized. However, the trend to relate allocations solely on the element of 'teaching' should be resisted and proper account taken of the contributions to postgraduate education, research training, and health research by the teaching hospitals; herein lies the future of good research and of a better health service.

It is important that the effect of reorganization of the NHS on teaching hospitals be carefully monitored. In Scotland, their support has now become the responsibility of the relevant area health board. It is understandable that the first responsibility of an AHB is for the service to its community and, with present financial constraints, a tendency to equate the claims of teaching and district hospitals can be appreciated. Conceding bias, I contend that this (if true) is a short-sighted policy and that the best interests of the NHS and of its growth and improvement depend more on the support of the growth points than on the spreading of available resources. It was the view of the Royal Commission on Medical Education (7) (para. 373) that

> the teaching hospital will always have special facilities which must be available to patients from outside its own district. The local population served by a single university teaching hospital will therefore be smaller than that served by an ordinary district hospital of the same size, but it must be sufficiently large and typical to provide opportunities for epidemiological research and for the teaching of community medicine.

Reorganization shows signs of producing yet another brake on research productivity. No one can deny that there has been multiplication of committees at hospital, district, area, and national levels and this has resulted in a growing demand on the time of senior clinical academic staff. Apart from the cost to the nation in terms of the time given by these individuals, together with growing travel expenses, this reduces the time which was formerly given either to research or to the supervision of research workers. It could be argued that as employees of the university these men have every opportunity to decline to participate in this overheated consultative machinery, but these are just the men who feel a responsibility to play their part in influencing decisions and the making of policy which affects the health service. And so, although clearly perceiving the dilemma, they usually decide to serve despite twinges of conscience at their diminishing commitment to research and patient care.

On a personal note, when first appointed consultant surgeon by the Western Regional Hospital Board to a teaching hospital (Western Infirmary, Glasgow) I was anxious to continue my clinical research interests. Thirty years ago, 'red tape' was more readily severed and without very much difficulty my full-time appointment was arranged so that seven sessions were the responsibility of the NHS and four sessions the responsibility of the MRC. I am well aware that this procedure has been repeated for external scientific staff to the MRC and that, occasionally, one or more research sessions have been included in a consultant's contract by the SHHD. However, this is the exception and usually results from a very specific request. I would like to see this type of contract being encouraged, particularly where the appointee is in an environment where research opportunity exists, and provided he has had a training which would fit him to use his special sessions profitably. This type of contract has been shown to benefit clinical research, and it could be an important means of encouraging and advancing health services research.

The universities and society. The discussion so far has centred around the problems facing universities at the present time, and the need to maintain their effective support. Universities too have many responsibilities and one of the greatest of these is to society.

For several centuries the universities have had patrons, but these were usually kings or merchant princes. Today they are obliged to accept block grants from the Treasury and so it must be recognized that it is the man in the street who is now the patron of learning. He is in a position to exercise the 'despotism of the majority' and that this has not been used so far is due, in large measure, to the protective role of the University Grants Committee. In its origins this was a simple device to keep government control at arm's length; it has proved to be a very effective mechanism and one which is envied by other countries. In effect parliament handed control over to a committee composed of men whose interests lay closer to the academic world than to the political world, and so those in control are in sympathy with those that are controlled. However the durability of this arrangement is open to question and the universities must constantly retain awareness of the need to adapt to their new patrons. This view is cogently argued by Ashby (8),

> but a university should interpret itself to its patrons and explain its need for autonomy. . . . The social institution which we call a university has endured now for seven centuries. It could have been destroyed, either by resisting pressure to change and so losing its viability, or by yielding too readily to change and so losing its integrity. But it has survived by adapting itself to the scientific revolution without abdicating its traditional functions in society. . . . The university is indeed an achievement of value, immensely worth preserving.

The time has come for the universities to adapt yet again to another revolution—the technicological one. Science has resided within the universities for centuries whereas technology is a relative newcomer which must be assimilated fully into academic life if the universities are to fulfil adequately their responsibility to society. Unlike science, which requires to work in a way which excludes variation from human judgement, technology is concerned with the applications of science to the needs of man and of society. The technologist, whether he likes it or not, cannot prevent himself from being involved in human problems. Medicine can be scientific but it is also one of the most ancient technologies; the medical research worker must concern himself not only with problems of a scientific nature but with some of the perpetual issues of humanity: family relationships, social justice, and ethics. In assimilating technology universities must steadily work towards the provision of an education which recognizes this. Whitehead (9), in *Science and the Modern World*, gives his views on the kind of adaptation which a university needs to make in order to assimilate technology:

there is something between the gross specialised values of the mere practical man, and the thin specialised values of the mere scholar. Both types have missed something; and if you add together the two sets of values, you do not obtain the missing element. When you understand all about the sun and all about the rotation of the earth, you may still miss the radiance of the sunset. There is no substitute for the direct perception of the concrete achievement of a thing in its actuality. . . . A factory, with its machinery, its community of operatives, its social service to the general population, its dependence upon organising and designing genius, its potentialities as a source of wealth to the holders of its stock is an organism exhibiting a variety of vivid values. What we want to train is the habit of apprehending such an organism in its completeness.

This is what society will expect higher education to achieve. It can be done through curricular changes provided these are not merely administrative but are accompanied by a change in academic attitudes.

Teachers of technology—in our context, teachers of medicine—will require to be convinced that the pattern of the curriculum under which they themselves were taught is inadequate for the new generation; teachers of arts will require to be persuaded that the presence of technology in universities puts them under an obligation to reconsider the exposition of their own humanistic studies. I do not doubt that, separately, both the technologies and the arts subjects are taught admirably but the time has come for an integration of their separate contributions and a joint appreciation of the necessary commitment of universities to society. They can no longer be independent of their new patron but they may continue to preserve autonomy by assuring the people of a strong and growing sense of responsibility to society. I use the words 'sense of responsibility' with care because the intellectual's concept of what society needs may differ from what society wants. Ashby (8) puts this dilemma succinctly:

they (the universities) are to-day regarded as popular national institutions, yet their activity sometimes obliges them to swim against the tide of popular opinion. Only by convincing their new patrons that they are working in the interests of society and not for themselves can they hope to preserve and consolidate that immunity from the despotism of the majority which they now enjoy. To do this requires delicate diplomacy. If universities were to become community service stations, responding to this and that popular demand, their integrity would be endangered and their influence weakened. If they were to become ivory towers, repudiating any responsibility to society, they would lose the confidence of their patrons.

I have suggested the need for changes in curricula but that this must be associated with changes in attitudes. I do not intend to invite criticism by making specific suggestions about curricular change in medical education, but elsewhere I have indicated the advantages of combined teaching. This technique could be used to liberalize medical education by involving teachers of sociology, political theory, moral philosophy, industrial psychology, etc. Whatever the courses devised, the subjects included should be taught in such a way to be directly relevant to the contemporary world and, in the broadest sense, to the technology of medicine.

In arguing the needs for adaptation, any implied criticism cannot detract from the enduring value of university achievement. Through their responsibility for research they have taken their place among the pacemakers for technological change; at a time when individuals are being pressed into uniformity by mass communication universities stand for the encouragement of variety, individuality, and preparedness to dissent. They have survived through the centuries by gradual adaptation and will do so again in a way which will be acceptable to the new patron and without abdicating traditional functions.

7

Communication with the public

There is much talk, and much is written, in these days about the importance of taking into account public or consumer opinion in determining policy relevant to public services; nowhere has this had a greater impact than in the field of health care. And yet, the concept of public opinion is both tenuous and elusive, and this is particularly so in the area of medicine where the level of consumer information and commitment is low. Furthermore, consumers of any public service rarely speak with a single voice; there are inevitable differences of interest; and so, sensible involvement in decision-making is difficult. How has the public's demand for involvement arisen? Can the public be meaningfully involved in the development of new policies? By what means can the public be given a coherent voice?

A brief glimpse back to the fourteenth century reminds us that about one-third of the population of Europe died within a single generation through total lack of knowledge concerning the cause of the Black Death. In the words of Sir Winston Churchill, 'it seemed to be the death-rattle of the race'. Even four centuries later the expectation of life was short and the picture was still one of survival of the fittest, and a fatalistic attitude still persisted. But now things began to change through the successes of science and technology, and it has become one of the anomalies of our time that the problems which we now face have resulted from these very successes; this applies in full measure to the improvements now available in health care.

There can be little doubt that the biological sciences, public health policies, and the influence of these on medical practice have led to remarkable progress in the prevention, control, and in some instances the curing of disease. Mortality rates have diminished and life expectancy has increased but in the wake of this success have come new problems such as population expansion and the growing need for care related to extended life-spans. The natural conditions of peoples' lives have been reshaped and a new environment has been created which offers unparalleled opportunities for life enrichment but, at the same time, we are living under the growing stress of continuing and accelerating change as a permanent condition of our lives and this we seem unable to control. Robert Burns, Scotland's national bard, celebrated in his poetry the value of goodness of simple things and I am sure that some would wish that our values could revert in this direction. But this cannot be and our task is to develop new concepts and new strategies for the control and solution of our problems. There is no choice but to try, and the task must be undertaken now. It is a daunting task and in the field of health we have much to learn. Our country is in a situation of debt which inevitably raises questions of the ultimate efficacy of government. Resultant inflation handicaps government's capacity to cope effectively with its wide range of responsibilities and it is tempted to seek solutions to problems through social and economic interventions which we fear may restrict both liberty and opportunity. We require a policy which is determined not by government alone but rather by the total attitude of our nation, including the attitudes and actions of individuals and groups.

This sketchy outline leading from public apathy to deep public concern leaves me in no doubt that the public must be meaningfully involved in present difficulties. It is therefore of the utmost importance to ensure that the public is informed in a responsible and unbiased way. The mass media provide a powerful instrument but at the present time much of the information provided is either inaccurate or skewed in a biased or emotive direction. This applies particularly to medical research and health care, on which further discussion is now focused.

Society will ask more and more questions about both the ends and means of health research. This means that attempts must be made to improve not only the partnership between government (as the formal representative of society) and the research community, but also between research centres (including hospitals) and their communities. This is important for the nation as a whole because sometimes government gets out of touch with the real needs and goals of society. Research workers who place their own self-interest ahead of the collective needs of medical research in society could be a problem for both the research community and the government. Participation in the public forum has important implications for our own social values as scientists. We should be fully aware of our responsibility to communicate with the public either through lay-type lectures, by greater and proper use of the mass media, and by contributions to semi-popular scientific journals; which ever medium is used, the scientist or teacher must adapt his presentations so that they are comprehensible to the audience. The Royal College of Physicians and Surgeons of Glasgow has, during the past few years, held interdisciplinary debates with representatives of other professions, giving consideration to such subjects as 'health in the permissive society'; the Colleges, through the President, have both the authority and opportunity to influence lay opinion by expressing considered views in the public press. There is also merit in Peart's (10) suggestion of a monthly forum on a question-and-answer basis, with an extension of the parliamentary select committee, involving the secretaries of the research councils and other major research trusts, scientists in appropriate fields and members of the press, and others who communicate with the public. 'Real initiative is necessary to get out of the cliché ridden atmosphere resounding with phrases like "ivory towers", "the faceless men of science" and "coldly scientific".' If medical research workers and medical practitioners are prepared to explain their ideas, their work, and their responsible intentions to the public I am confident that they will be fully accepted as a vital element in the fabric of society.

In order to communicate meaningfully and successfully with the public the medical research community must express its sense of responsibility and reaffirm its traditional image as a profession that cares. I believe that a declaration of this sort is a matter of urgency at this time when some life and death issues are becoming—perhaps unfortunately—matters for public debate. Two examples will suffice: euthanasia and terminal care which, largely through medical and technological advances, present new dilemmas.

Euthanasia is described in the dictionary as 'mercy killing', but it would be more accurate to call it 'therapeutic murder'. It is based on the philosophy that what is useful is right. If one can destroy the dying patient to relieve his pain, one can put him to death like a sick animal; he can be killed just because he is a burden to his family and to society. As Dunphy (11) has pointed out:

> in Nazi Germany the opening wedge for mass genocide was the presentation to the public of films illustrating how gently and beautifully life could be taken from a patient because he was crippled, incompetent, or suffering. This was the first step. The next was the elimination of the life of anyone who gave someone else a sense of being pained, uncomfortable, or burdened. Justified by Hegelian philosophy, mercy killing of the sick and incompetent by deliberate and positive actions paved the way to the gas chamber for millions of innocent men, women, and children.

The moral question for members of the medical profession is not whether the suffering and the dying are persons, but whether *we* are the kind of persons who will care for them without doubting their worth. We cannot destroy life and must state this categorically. If there are those in our society who think otherwise, let them work for a totalitarian form of government where euthanasia for the infirm and incompetent has led to its use for the intellectually dissident. The care of the hopelessly ill or mentally deficient is a taxing but noble burden that the health professions have assumed through the years and must proclaim their willingness to continue to bear.

A very fine but critical line exists between a positive action that leads to death (euthanasia) and the withholding or withdrawing of forms of treatment which prolong life without benefiting the patient: 'finer and harder to see than the Thin Red Line of Balaclava it is of immensely greater importance that it be held for the preservation of morality and life in this small world'. It is my personal belief that it is wrong to resuscitate the terminal patient, to prolong a useless and tragic life by parenteral feeding, or to frustrate pneumonia—the friend of the hopelessly ill and lonely aged—by the giving of antibiotics. It is inhuman to give chemotherapy or radiation therapy to the dying cancer patient if all the 'treatment' offers is a dragging out of an intolerable existence for a few more agonizing days or weeks. The secret of the care of the patient is in truly caring for that patient and without 'caritas' the public would lose confidence in, and be unlikely to communicate freely with, the medical researcher and the practitioner. The proper care of the dying patient does not end with the withdrawal of special forms of treatment. Skilled nursing care, appropriate relief of pain and, more importantly, regular thoughtful visits by all members of the caring team may not prolong life but will permit death with comfort and dignity. It is my experience that the patient who is near unto death is not afraid of death, but he is very much afraid of being abandoned by his doctor in the face of death.

In these two examples lies the most important information which the medical profession should communicate to the public —at individual doctor/patient level and at a campaign level— namely, that we understand, that we care and that we will always care. This would go a long way towards relieving public anxiety because implicit in this would be an affirmation of the sense of responsibility which doctors will exercise in advancing research in medicine.

As an addendum, it should not go without note that the ability of medicine to prolong life by artificial means has attracted the attention not only of the public but of the legal profession. The Karen Ann Quinlan case highlights this issue and doctors would do well to heed the warning of Richard A. McCormick (12) in a recent Editorial in the *Journal of the American Medical Association*:

> The real moral issue in the Quinlan case is not merely a narrowly casuistic one but the limits of our duty to sustain life. That problem is present, of course, but the abiding issue is deeper and broader than that. It is the very moral matrix of the healing profession. That matrix roots in the conviction that decision-making within health care, if it is to remain truly human and an expression of the cardinal rule of the physician, *primum non nocere*, must be controlled primarily within the patient–doctor–family relationship, and these decisions must be tailor-made to individual cases and circumstances. If technology and law were largely to usurp these prerogatives—as they threaten to do as a result of the Quinlan case—we would all be worse off; impersonal considerations would replace personal ones and preprogram our treatment. That is always the route of oppression and depersonalisation, in medicine as well as in economics, government, and the church; . . .

On the assumption that mutual confidence has again been firmly established let us consider a few of the many issues on which the public should be informed and involved. First, people have tended to be blinded by the brilliant achievements of medical research during the past thirty or forty years and so have failed to realize that medical treatment has its limitations. The cause, and therefore cure, of such diseases as cancer and rheumatoid arthritis cannot be provided by science merely for the asking nor by the injection of massive finance. The fruits of recent research have led to a general desire to want more and to have better, but it is essential to modify immediate expectations; 'more' and 'better' are not always the same, and more now is not always compatible with the objective of more later. People are capable of discerning where their real interest lies but choice is involved and for this sound information must be provided, both sides of a question must always be presented, and at all times truth is of the essence.

Secondly, in contrast to the first, we must find more effective methods of informing the public about the availability of the health care services, that their existence has so far not guaranteed their proper use, that they are over-used by some and, more importantly, under-used by many.

Thirdly, the second leads to a realization of our present failure to impress upon people their personal responsibility for preventing ill health. This despite the excellent endeavours of the health educationalist. In this regard it is perhaps somewhat discouraging to appreciate that the campaign towards promoting personal health was supported in telling fashion by Dr John Brown (13), a medical practitioner of the latter half of the last century. In a charming essay on 'Health' he wrote:

My dear friends,—I am going to give you a sort of sermon about your health, —and you know a sermon has always a text; so, though I am only a doctor, I mean to take a text of ours, and I will choose it, as our good friends the ministers do, from the best of all books, the Bible. Job ii. 4: 'All that a man hath will he give for his life'.

If you had £500 in a box at home, and knew that you would certainly be dead by to-morrow unless you gave the £500, would you ever make a doubt about what you would do? Not you! And if you were told that if you got drunk, or worked too hard, or took no sort of care of your bodily health, you would turn ill to-morrow and die next week, would you not keep sober, and work more moderately, and be more careful of yourself?

Now, I want to make you believe that you are too apt to do this very same sort of thing in your daily life, only that instead of to-morrow or next week, your illness and your death comes next year or, at any rate, some years sooner than otherwise. But your death is actually preparing already, and that by your own hands, by your own ignorance, and often by your own foolish and sinful neglect and indulgence.

Dr Brown defined disease as the opposite of health and preached that it will come to us by descent from our parents, by excessive work (and here he referred to occupational diseases), excessive pleasures and ignorance of the laws of health; the latter he defined as those plain common things which, if we do we will live long, and which, if we do not do, we will die earlier. The people in our day have been informed but behaviour has not changed markedly; communication must continue until they are convinced.

Fourthly, another issue to which we should turn our attention before it becomes a major one in this country is the value of a routine annual medical physical examination—already a major issue in the USA. After reviewing the information provided by the Kaiser Permanente programme Dr Richard Spark of Harvard, quoted in the *New York Times*, posed this question: 'Why do people who submit to these periodic examinations have the same disease disability and mortality rate as those who seek medical advice only when they feel sick?' I would wish to counter this by yet another question, namely, 'is there hard evidence for the above statement?' If there is, and we add the acknowledged risk of engendering an introspective attitude by regular medical examination, the procedure should not be encouraged; if on the other hand the statement is ill-founded, soundly planned studies are required to provide an informed answer. We are not without opportunity in this country for planning such studies because annual medical examinations are increasingly used by various industrial organizations. Society will make the demand; let research be ready with the evidence.

Finally, one of the most pressing problems facing medicine today is the escalation of medical costs and the effects that this will have on the provision of services to the public, and on the professional lives of doctors. Society should be made aware of the problem and the part research can play in its solution. Most countries, including the United Kingdom, enjoyed a steady growth of health services after the Second World War. The public, increasingly impressed with the seemingly unending achievements of medicine, has developed an almost insatiable appetite for health services. Some limitation of services is inevitable and this must be recognized by all. Government is paying the bills for health care and, whether we like it or not, it is incumbent upon the profession to be able to answer questions posed by government and it must play its own part in tackling the problem. Faced with this challenge and forced to accept a painful slowing down of resources, does the profession find itself in a state of preparedness?

Traditionally, doctors have been concerned mainly with the sick and the injured (and this at an individual level), have thought little in terms of groups of patients, and practically not at all about the cost of medical care. If the demand for services is unlimited and resources limited, the solution is no longer simply a social issue but also an economic one. Medicine alone cannot provide the solutions and society must face up to some agonizing decisions as to how health care money can best be spent; however, a considerable burden of responsibility rests with the medical profession. I suggest that 'medicine' must recapture the quality of community leadership that has been a part of its heritage, and unless doctors become as concerned about the costs of medical care as they have tried to be about its quality, the fulfilment of the public's wants may all too soon become an externally imposed reality.

It is important that we identify the kind of 'medical care' which represents the major burden on the health care system. Is this not the management of those diseases for which we are as yet unable to offer any definitive therapy or prevention, and so we offer affected patients what has been called 'the half-way medical technologies'? This is the best we can do for patients who have diseases which we have not the knowledge to prevent but for which we have developed supportive measures. It is not so long ago that this was all we could offer the patient suffering from poliomyelitis, and at that time the cost of supportive therapy for such a patient would probably surpass that of the present-day treatment of a patient requiring haemodialysis for chronic renal failure. Similarly, the acute nutritional and vitamin deficiencies have disappeared from the Western world, and it would not be difficult to reel off many disorders which we have now brought under control with definitive therapy and prevention so that they no longer make major demands upon our resources. There remains a long list of diseases which reflect our ignorance of their causation and management and I venture to predict that each will pass through a phase in which the supportive measures will become increasingly 'successful' but increasingly costly. Our main hope in solving this problem is to seek with increased vigour the knowledge and understanding which will lead to rational preventive or therapeutic procedures. Success cannot be guaranteed but if we do not pursue this course unconquered diseases will continue to take their toll, and will continue to confront society with the dilemma of deciding the amount of the nation's resources given to health care.

In the short term, society should be aware that doctors are now taking a growing interest in conserving resources required for the cost of medical care; in the long term, society should appreciate that the solution will come from fundamental exploratory research which must be given adequate support and must not be penalized by an excessive diversion of resources to operational research. Balance must be preserved and research in medicine must advance on a broad front.

8

Career prospects in medical research

Important though adequate financial provision is for the furtherance of medical research, in the ultimate, progress will depend on the skills and sound training of scientists. The maintenance of a cadre of trained research workers of high quality is therefore of prime importance.

During the period of steady financial growth the careers of research workers was not a serious problem: some gained a tenured appointment with a research council or similar organization, while others gained academic posts in universities. However, the effect of the transition from continuous growth to a steady state has altered this situation; translation to established university posts has been severely limited. Again, most research workers are not a race apart and like individuals in other sectors of the community have a reasonable desire to achieve the security of a tenured appointment at a rather earlier age than was customary up until the end of the 1960s; they get married, they have mortgages and they have families to educate.

This growing problem was given special consideration by the MRC when it held its first ever Council meeting out of London, in the University of Edinburgh in November 1975. Members of Council had the opportunity to meet officers of the University, together with representatives of other Scottish universities. The Nuffield Provincial Hospitals Trust has also taken an initiative with particular reference to the training and tenure of research workers in the field of health services research and several meetings have been held with health department representatives to focus on this problem. I have attended these, and other meetings at which this subject has been under discussion, and have at all times gained the impression that there was much greater success in highlighting the difficulties than in providing constructive ideas

TABLE 3. *Staff employed at 1 January 1973, 1976, and 1977*

Category of Staff	*Total*			*Secretary of State*			*SHERT*		
	1973	*1976*	*1977*	*1973*	*1976*	*1977*	*1973*	*1976*	*1977*
Professional scientific	49	40	30	38	30	20	11	10	10
Medical *without* honorary clinical contract	6	2	–	6	1	–	–	1	–
Medical *with* honorary clinical contract	22	8	9	15	6	5	7	2	4
Technicians	45	32	30	35	22	17	10	10	13
Others	16	6	2	14	5	1	2	1	1
Total	138	88	71	108	64	43	30	24	28

towards solutions. This is not a reflection on the organization of the meetings, nor should it deter us from grasping instead of grappling with the problem.

It is generally held at this time that there has been a decline in medical research within universities but there is a lack of hard information. The secretariat of BRC, at the request of the Committee, produced data on the staff employed at 1 January 1973, 1976, and 1977 (Table 3) which revealed that there has been a marked decline in the number of medically qualified staff who have been funded on research grants over this period. There are good reasons for encouraging a promising medical or dental graduate to learn research skills early in his postgraduate career and to gain experience in a selected area of investigation related to the study of disease, the preservation of health, the care of the sick, or provision of health services; this fall-off is disturbing and merits careful monitoring. Does the change reflect a gradual decline and will it continue? Will a steady state develop, or can a period of renewed growth be anticipated?

In attempting to dissect the career prospects of research workers in medicine it is necessary to consider clinical and non-clinical staff separately; the latter are numerically greater and, in addition, they encounter greater difficulties in changing to a career other than research.

Medically qualified research workers. The problem for members of this group is that there are now real disincentives to the pursuit of research training or a career in research, and this in turn raises anxieties concerning the future of the nation's capacity for research related to medicine.

Formerly, medical graduates who had proceeded to gain a research training soon after graduation formed the group from which junior appointments were made to MRC Unit establishments or to clinical and science academic departments. The second alternative has been made difficult by the present financial stringencies affecting the universities together with the fact that teaching has priority over research in the allocation of resources. Despite limited opportunity for choosing an academic career, there will continue to be a small but important group of doctors who are determined to pursue research irrespective of this barrier, financial reward, or conditions of service. Potentially, these are the 'high fliers' and merit encouragement: although some will be successful in gaining a research council training award, others are in danger of being committed to a successive research-grant-assisted life which even the most enthusiastic researcher is liable to find incompatible with the level of family life now demanded by other sectors of society. Fortunately, from the young man's viewpoint, he has much safer career alternatives; research in medicine is the loser. The man can opt to take a junior appointment in the NHS, thereby augmenting his salary, follow the path of his main clinical interest and work towards the acquisition of the appropriate college diploma. Again, a decision to translate to general practice would be an even more speedy route towards financial security. A research interest and some training is also an advantage in seeking a career in the administrative side of the NHS or in the pharmaceutical industry.

Maintenance of recruitment of medical graduates to research is hindered severely by two major changes which have taken place during the past decade: the increased rigidity of specialist training programmes, and the introduction of new arrangements for paying junior hospital staff.

In the recent past, when a hospital consultant's training could take about ten years, active participation of a junior graduate in research projects could accelerate his progress towards a consultant post. With the introduction of the fairly rigid training programmes over a seven-year period, the completion of which will almost ensure a consultancy, it is apparent that even a short period in research will add substantially to the time a trainee would take to reach his career post. While I concede that the training programmes may have raised the general standard of surgery, medicine, etc., the end-products have been prepared in a common mould and there is no encouragement for the individualist. In the west of Scotland we are fortunate that the Postgraduate Committee in Surgery allows a more flexible course of training for lecturers in surgery who have been given honorary status as senior registrars; unfortunately, the restricted allocation of honorary senior registrar posts is such that about half the lecturers in my discipline, although possessing the FRCS diploma and having completed acceptable training at junior level, are not able to be enrolled in Higher Surgical Training. Despite this, their training proceeds in a similar manner to their fellows in the NHS and, in addition, they have increased responsibility for teaching and time has to be found for their contribution to the academic department's research programme. The demands put on these men are greater, progress to consultant status is delayed until they gain promotion to senior lectureship level, and should they fail to gain this academic promotion those who did not have the benefit of honorary senior registrar status will have to spend additional time satisfying the somewhat rigid criteria of higher training programmes. Although an improvement in training was recommended by the Royal Commission on Medical Education this inflexibility was not intended. Let me recall some of the paragraphs of the RCME Report (7). From paragraph 76 come these words

> during the three years of general professional training young doctors should be allowed, if they show the aptitude, to undertake worthwhile research *without being penalised financially*; if a trainee spent part of his general professional training period in approved full-time research, he should be allowed to pursue his research interest thereafter on a part-time basis. Any research done should be taken fully into account in the assessment at the end of the period. We hope very much that any who show enthusiasm and ability for research will be encouraged to begin some original work at this stage: new ideas and quests for fresh horizons are essentially qualities of youth.

Towards the end of paragraph 93: 'if, as we hope, the early postgraduate phase ceases to be dominated by preparation for formal examinations, many more trainees than at present should be able to take part in research'. Finally, in paragraph 109:

> the present senior registrar training schemes have been improved as the result of the establishment of advisory committees jointly by universities and hospital authorities, but there is still a good deal to be done, particularly in providing a variety of experience and opportunities for research. At present few senior registrars get any real opportunity to carry out clinical research, as is shown by the fact that few obtain a higher degree in the course of their training. This is a serious defect in the education of those who will eventually carry the most responsible and influential posts in medicine and steps should be taken to remedy it. We hope that a substantial proportion of those selected for intensive training posts will obtain a higher degree in the course of their training.

While it must be admitted that a year of training can be spent in research under the new regulations, this provides merely 'a look at research'; it does not provide a research training and fortunate will be the man who gains a higher degree on the basis of one year's work on a research project. There can be little doubt that the 'safe' course for a young graduate to pursue in these days is to proceed as quickly as he can through junior to higher training and thereby take the shortest possible route to a consultant post.

I do not advocate that all should spend an appreciable time in research; this is for those with a real interest. Again, my own experience leads me to believe that a minority only of medical graduates who spend a year or more in research proceed to become dedicated scientists or prosper in academic medicine. Hopefully, however, the others will acquire a questioning and critical attitude which will influence beneficially their subsequent professional practice, and some will continue to be involved in clinical or health services research and, as their laboratories will be the hospital wards or the local community, they can do this even in these days of financial restriction. These men have much to offer in raising the standard of clinical practice in district hospitals. Sadly, I have had several experiences on appointment committees where local members openly stated that a research training was not desirable and that a curriculum vitae containing several good scientific publications, while perhaps of help in gaining a consultant post in a teaching hospital, had little meaning for the post under consideration. These attitudes militate strongly against the national move towards the upgrading of the 'non-teaching' hospitals and the over-all improvement of the health service throughout our country.

It can be concluded that, conceding their contribution to a good level of medical care, the relative inflexibility of training programmes places a low value on research training and encourages the safe and quickest route to a career consultant post. But, more recently, there has been a further discouragement for young men with an interest in medical research.

The new arrangements for paying junior hospital staff for duties in excess of the basic working week have now led to a situation where a substantial part of a doctor's salary (up to about £2,000) can come in a form of 'overtime payments'. It is evident that there is a financial disincentive for a junior hospital doctor to being employed through a research support grant, even if he does not lose in hierarchical status. In my own view the acceptance of this arrangement will do irreparable harm to the ethos of medicine and is already reducing the momentum of all aspects of research in medicine. As I write, UMTs are being paid regularly to junior hospital doctors on NHS contracts while their counterparts in clinical academic departments have been without this substantial salary increment since October 1976; I am not aware of the reasons for withholding these payments to clinical lecturers but it is presumably related to indecision about determining the paymaster—the NHS, since the payments are for additional clinical care?—the universities from existing financial allocations? —the universities through special additional allocations from the UGC? Hopefully, the payments will be made retrospectively to men who have previously undertaken mortgages and other similar family responsibilities but, in the meantime, the situation is bound to reflect adversely on recruitment to clinical and paraclinical departments.[1] It is my fervent, but perhaps futile, hope that we can return to paying hospital doctors in our NHS a salary for the job, that the salary will be comparable with that received by our colleagues in other countries, and that we will care for the individual patients for whom we are responsible at all times of the day or night without any consideration for

1. UMTs now paid to junior academic clinicians.

additional payments. I believe that this view would be upheld by many in the medical profession, perhaps particularly in Scotland where the majority devote their full time to the NHS, and it is to be hoped that the health departments will not too readily agree to a continuance of extra duty payments to junior hospital doctors and progression to a similar arrangement for consultant staff. Continued moves in this direction would militate against the avowed wish of the health departments to encourage a growing interest in all aspects of medical research and, in particular, health services research.

The major problems have been outlined and some solutions inferred. First, there is a need for increased flexibility in the training programmes supervised by the specialist advisory committees. Secondly, the serious effects of the extra duty payment system are already evident, not on research only but on many aspects of medical care, and it is to be hoped that the Royal Commission will consider this in the course of its work. Thirdly, it is important that a proportion, albeit quite small, of medical graduates be encouraged to undertake an extensive course of research training and it is for the research councils, the health departments, and other major granting authorities to ensure that this can be done. The solution will not be easy and it will be expensive and may require the institution of long-term training awards leading to a tenured post in some discipline of medical research. Fourthly, it is argued by some that the present method of funding a medical graduate for scientific training immediately after the pre-registration posts is inadvisable, and that the young man would be better advised to postpone research experience until after the acquisition of a College diploma since this is an essential step in a young consultant's career. Those subscribing to this viewpoint would advocate the institution of senior research fellowships funded at the post-diploma level. For myself, I believe that the earlier a young clinician receives research training the better. The younger a man is, the more easily can he accept new material which is conceptually difficult. Most subjects in the medical course are not intellectually difficult to assimilate, but the sheer volume of knowledge which must be covered by the student is formidable. On the other hand, many scientific concepts are difficult to understand, especially those with a mathematical basis, and the younger a man is when he tackles them the better. This is becoming more and more clear as the biological sciences become increasingly dependent on a knowledge of physics, chemistry, and mathematics. If the young doctor spends several years in vocational training he may well be in his late twenties or early thirties before he has time for scientific training; to return at this stage to the study of basic scientific principles is not easy. I fully realize that I make my plea for an early introduction to research techniques in difficult days. Formerly, the Medical Research Council provided adequately funded scholarships for training in research methods for both medical and science graduates who wished to continue training in the medical field beyond the first degree. Medical graduates who had completed their pre-registration hospital appointments may also gain Council's Junior Research Fellowships which are tenable either in the department in which the candidate is already working or at other suitable centres in the United Kingdom. The Council also awards fellowships in clinical research to medical graduates who wish to study methods of research in the basic subject most relevant to their particular clinical interest and to broaden their experience by working in other departments either in their own university or elsewhere in the UK. However, while postgraduate scientific training continues to be available through such awards, applicants are now penalized in terms of finance or of prospects for promotion. Fortunately there will always be the very few who are sufficiently strongly motivated to be prepared to work and persevere despite the penalties, but is this the way to encourage research which has as its objective the steady improvement of the nation's health service?

THE NON-CLINICAL SCIENTIST

In the 1960s the science graduate wishing to pursue a research career had, as one of several alternatives, employment in the steadily expanding universities. At that time a 'research group' or 'research unit' was established within a university on condition that the university would accept financial responsibility at the end of a stated number of years. Today a university can rarely accept responsibility for such a 'take-over' arrangement. And yet the nation, with the help of the universities, needs to ensure the existence of a corps of experienced researchers trained to study biomedical, clinical, and health service problems. It is evident that a career structure, and improved career prospects, have become an urgent requirement.

Proposals to meet this need should take cognizance of the fact that scientists vary in talents and abilities and so the methods of support will also vary. Junior, untenured, research staff fall into three broad categories. The first group consists of the highly qualified scientists who can be expected to achieve, even in times of financial constraint, academic tenure or tenure as leading scientists with a research council. They will be few in number, will usually be identified as they approach their late twenties, and do not constitute a major problem. However, it is important to provide support for these individuals until scientific potential is proven and tenure can be offered. One safeguard for a young scientist between the ages of 20–30 could be through the establishment of a fellowship scheme agreed by a university and a research council, or, in the case of health services research, by a health department and a university. While the authorities concerned would be jointly interested in the trainee's career and eventual posting, the financial responsibility would rest with the research council or with the health department. In this way the university entering into the agreement would be strengthened for a period of up to ten years by the fellow's research contribution; the research council (or the health authority) would be promoting mobility and mutual exchange of ideas with the university and on conclusion of the Fellowship one or other would take the Fellow on to its permanent staff. The number of Fellowships to be awarded would need careful consideration so that the organizations concerned would be able to absorb the 'graduates' without detriment to undertakings for existing staff. It would seem, therefore, that a solution for this first group of recruits to research is feasible provided the authorities concerned are willing to share responsibility and absorb approximately equal numbers of 'graduates' from the fellowship scheme.

The second group of young scientists are those with specialized scientific skills who would not normally achieve academic tenure in the university department to which they were attached, but bring to that department skills which enlarge its research capability. The training of these men is usually different from the central discipline of that department, for example, a biochemist in an academic department of surgery or an electron microscopist in a department of dermatology; they play a very important role in providing a service to research. I would also include in this category scientists capable of acting as second-in-command to a professor, or to a director of a research unit. He has a wide experience of research and is able to cope effectively with the day-to-day problems posed by junior staff, but he depends for the direction of the research on the departmental head. These individuals are invaluable to senior academics wishing to continue in research despite large external claims on their time. When men possessing these qualities emerge they should be encouraged, since they probably constitute one of the most efficient ways of providing research support. The securement of posts for the two types of scientists in my second group are at the present time increasingly beyond the means of universities. This is not through financial stringency alone but also because the UGC uses the student/staff ratio as the main criterion for the allocation of grants to universities, thereby effectively inhibiting the appointment of research staff. The essential preliminary to securing the employment of these scientists is the recognition that they have much to offer each and every university. The next step is the recognition by individual university departments that they must be prepared to make a contribution towards the solution of this problem. In the absence of these assurances it would be unreasonable to expect a research council or a health department to accept long-term commitments for such staff. However if it is recognized that individuals with specialized expertise can be of great assistance to several departments within a university, and that their skills can be deployed among these departments, the university authorities can insist on the need for collaboration of all science and medical departments to maintain and supervise this category through some central machinery. The time is ripe for universities to consider the feasibility of this proposition.

The third category of research workers are usually on short-term contracts, typically of three years' duration. They are salaried by research grants and are usually in their early twenties. This is not usually a problem category but within the group there may be 'the lad o' pairts' who, when identified, merits consideration for longer-term support to prove his ability for inclusion in the first group.

In considering this urgent and taxing problem of career opportunities required to ensure the maintenance of a body of experienced research workers, some important principles should influence policy definition. First, there must be opportunity for the individual worker to improve his abilities and pursue his personal ambitions. This implies that any plan should have a flexibility which will enable staff to transfer easily once a department's research has been completed or is no longer relevant. Secondly, an essential requirement for appointments to a tenured post must be acceptable evidence of ability either as an original worker, or as an individual with a particular skill to offer to a research team. It may take up to ten years to assess the former, and somewhat less for the latter. In order to ensure the best appointments to a system of tenured posts selection should be by competition. Thirdly, a researcher accepting a tenured appointment should also accept the principle of redeployment if required. Thus, as far as health services research is concerned, workers should be prepared to move into service or administrative work within the NHS or take teaching posts in relevant university departments. It should be understood that when there is need to redeploy a research worker it may not be possible to find a suitable post in the nearby area, and so the policy based on these principles must be of a national character.

Throughout this discussion I have referred particularly to the relationship between the research council organizations and the universities but most is relevant to the relationship between the health departments and the universities especially in relation to clinical and health services research. For almost a decade the health departments have been committed to support research designed to improve the service, and the establishment of Chief Scientist Organizations underlines this commitment. Whereas the research councils must be concerned to maintain a research capacity in the biomedical field, the health departments face the task of building, and thereafter maintaining a health services research capacity. To achieve this aim I suggest that the health departments will require to enter into an arrangement with universities of the dual support type which is at the centre of research council policy.

9

Implementation of research results

More than one interpretation has been put on the words of Lord Rosenheim, made during an address to the World Health Organization in 1968: 'If, for the next twenty years no further research were to be carried out, if there were a moratorium on research, the application of what is already known, of what has already been discovered would result in widespread improvement in world health.' Dr John Brown, a medical practitioner who worked in the latter half of the last century, and best known through such delightful essays as *Rab and his Friends*, expressed a similar thought in his *Horae Subsecivae* in 1886: 'the great thing in regulating and benefiting human life is not to find out new things, but to make the best of the old things'. It is my view that Lord Rosenheim was not advocating a stop to research in medicine, but highlighting failure to implement accepted research results particularly in deprived countries throughout the world. Correction of this failure has not yet been achieved and this was emphasized by Dr Mahler, Director-General of WHO in his address to the 29th Assembly in 1976:

> We have witnessed in this century extraordinary advances in science and technology which have been applied to the prevention and treatment of disease, and the rehabilitation of the disabled and infirm. The pace of this progress has accelerated enormously in the past quarter century. However, its fruits have been enjoyed by a relatively small proportion of the world's population. We are still seeking by hard scientific endeavour to unravel the mysteries of some of the most serious health scourges of mankind. The desire to discover is insatiable, and in itself it is probably laudable; but we cannot stop at mere discovery. Technology for the sake of technology is a dangerous addiction-producing drug. We must always bear in mind the practical application of existing and new scientific knowledge for the benefit of the masses of the world's population. Here lies the challenge.

This is one facet of implementation of research results but, important though it is, it is not my intention to consider it further here.

Nor will I discuss in any detail the dissemination and implementation of the results of basic research and the more fundamental studies in clinical research. It is a characteristic of this type of research that success lies in the past and in the future, but not in the present. Scientists alone have a full appreciation of the amount of work, often in a variety of disciplines, which is required before there is full development of usable knowledge. As far as the layman is concerned the introduction of a major therapeutic advance is regarded as a sudden 'breakthrough' which will soon be taken for granted. The scientific steps leading to the development of penicillin, the oral contraceptive pill, and chemotherapy began more than a century before they were introduced. The summation of these steps ultimately led to the major advances. Mustard (6) refers to this as the 'paradox of time':

> the paradox of time is that society cannot easily recognise what is being done now, as a base for future success, and will readily forget past successes as well as what went into making them possible. This paradox of time makes research support from a public purse vulnerable to being forgotten in the political process, particularly when there is pressure on the use of public funds.

It will continue to be the responsibility of scientists to appraise each new gain in knowledge and relate this to similar gains in fields other than their own so that a considered judgement on their significance can be made. However, despite the ease with which the results of research can be published in specialized journals, difficulties in communication between scientists from different disciplines persists. Despite growing demand for multidisciplinary research, it is often surprisingly difficult even to get basic scientists and clinicians together and many opportunities for fruitful research are thereby lost. The astute clinician has no difficulty in defining neglected areas but either fails to pass this information on to the appropriate scientist, or fails to appreciate the importance of doing so. The communication problem between scientists of differing disciplines, and between scientists and doctors, is another major challenge. It could, to some extent, be met by much greater selectivity and discrimination on the part of publishers or those supporting publication; there are too many papers based on 'nit-picking' as opposed to forward-looking research. An alternative, with even greater merit, would be more critical comment from an alert scientific community.

There is yet another challenge, which is my main concern at this time, and this is the implementation of results from the more applied end of the research spectrum: health services research and applied clinical research. Here again it must be admitted that there is no well-defined policy for the application of new knowledge and information. Again, the basic defect is the lack of effective communication between researchers, those who plan and conduct the service, and those giving the service. Resources spent on research and development will be wasted unless communication is improved and the research organization backed up by effective machinery for passing on the results to the individuals at the sharp end of the exercise. The broad climate of opinion at a particular time is of the utmost importance, as is the ability to influence all involved within the service. It follows from this that the 'top of the office' in the health departments must not merely communicate but work in a collaborative exercise with the researchers and with all members of the caring professions; there is room for optimism that this can be achieved in the longer term as a consequence of the reorganization which has taken place in our National Health Service, provided that the organization can develop an increased capacity for adaptation and change, together with a sharpened ability to focus on the innovations which are likely to be most beneficial.

While I hesitate to attempt the formulation of a policy for the implementation of research results I am prepared to make suggestions which, if themselves implemented, may go some way towards improving the present situation.

The usual method of communicating the results of medical research is through medical and scientific journals but, unless aided by review articles and leaders, it is often difficult to discriminate between significant and unimportant advances. Furthermore, I suspect that the journals are scrutinized by a minority, scanned by others, and filed for 'future reading' by many. In any event, no one doctor could read them all and the more specialized journals are of interest mainly to those in the relevant discipline. Although a vast amount of information produced weekly can be analysed and presented by the Medlars system or the cumulative *Index Medicus* these tend to be used mainly by researchers when planning projects or reviewing the literature for manuscript preparation. And so it seems to me that this form of communication is inadequate to meet the objective of implementing the results of research—with one exception. The *Health Bulletin*, which is issued by the Chief Medical Officer of the Scottish Home and Health Department and includes reports from the Chief Scientist, goes some way towards filling the need. It is circulated, without charge, to medical and dental practitioners and certain other health care workers throughout Scotland. This under-rated, under-priced, and I suspect inadequately read monthly publication provides a continuing commentary on research in progress, completed research, health education, and almost all aspects of the service at work; in addition, there are contributions from research workers, from staff in the hospital service, and from general practitioners. If communication by way of the written word can be effective this type of publication provides a medium for success.

Medical education should provide an excellent method of communicating the significant results of research, of preparing the climate of professional opinion, and of encouraging the translation of new ideas into service. This should begin at the undergraduate level where the opportunity should be grasped to indicate trends, stimulate interest in fields which are ripe for development, and instil the concept that research without implementation of its beneficial results is a luxury in our time. The need for continuing education after graduation is now generally accepted and the growing number of postgraduate medical teaching centres, for long a priority area for support by the Nuffield Provincial Hospitals Trust, should play an important role. However, my own experience is that implementation of research to influence change within the service has had low priority. Most programmes are built around a series of formal lectures, given by eminent clinicians or distinguished research workers, which are liable to leave the audience with the problem of evaluating the substance of the lecture. The heavily committed practitioner of medicine has a right to expect that much of the evaluation will be prepared for him, the defects in current practice clearly spelt out, and improvement trends indicated. I do not belittle the considerable achievements of continuing education in the last two decades but there is now a need to recognize its potential as a means of disseminating medical information and of hastening the introduction of desirable changes in the NHS. The importance of social contact and informal discussion within those postgraduate centres which are a focal point for the meeting of consultants, family doctors, and community physicians should not be ignored; this will lead to better collaboration, a fuller mutual understanding of health service problems, and real involvement.

The Royal Colleges have a unique opportunity, and indeed a great responsibility, to improve communication within the profession. For centuries the Colleges have upheld standards in individual patient care and this should now embrace a responsibility for the standard of health service offered to the public. Traditionally, each College has tended to act mainly on behalf of its own membership; recent moves towards unified action are welcome and urgently needed. The Royal Colleges and Faculties, which are national bodies independent of governmental control, must preserve and use their power to speak clearly and forcibly in the interests of our patients and our professional standards. An important step towards collaboration was taken in Scotland in April 1973, when the first meeting was held of the Joint Conference of Colleges and Faculties within Scotland. This has since been followed by a similar development in England and Wales and arrangements have been made for at least annual meetings of the two Joint Conferences. The Colleges can play a major role in implementing the results of research within the service by moving outward into the district, organizing symposia in selected geographical areas and doing this in a collaborative way by nominating a representative from each College and Faculty to attend. Conference material should include such topics as quality of care, medical audit, controlled trials resulting in a clear outcome, optimum use of acute surgical beds, utilization of services, etc.; for most, presentation of the results of surveys, clinical trials, and experiments should be a central feature. Although efforts of this sort will not set the Health Service right tomorrow, they will influence opinions, attitudes, and ambitions.

In the last ten years the Colleges have organized and taken responsibility for the overview of specialist training programmes. Although in large measure beneficial, I have referred elsewhere to the real danger of rigidity interfering with the research training of young men. In addition to encouraging a more flexible attitude in this regard, I would like to see an authoritative statement to the effect that sound training and publications in health services research are as acceptable as in biomedical research. The inclusion of examination questions relating to controlled trials, etc., would ensure that future diplomates recognized their importance. Finally, most of the Royal Colleges inform their Fellows and Members through journals or bulletins and here again is an opportunity to influence attitudes within the profession.

The development of a policy for implementing the results of research should take into account the potential benefits offered by two important organizational changes in the service in recent years: the 'Cogwheel' divisional structure, and the National Medical Consultative Committee with its specialty sub-committees. With regard to the former I fully recognize that the main objective was to encourage clinicians to participate in management and to convince them that this was essential to the interests of their patients and to the proper position of their profession. A survey of the reaction to 'Cogwheel' was made by the Nuffield Provincial Hospitals Trust in 1971 (14), but this now requires updating and the provision of a report on the successes and the failures, with the reasons for each outcome. It is even more important today for clinicians to appreciate that if they do not accept responsibility for the planning and management of the service to their patients, the opportunity to do so may slip away, together with their ability to influence their own affairs. However my interest at this time is in the use of the divisional structure to encourage research and assist in the implementation of worthwhile results. Here should originate randomized controlled trials because involvement of all clinicians within the division ensures an adequate intake to the trial; again, participation in the planning and conduct of the trial would go a long way to ensure implementation at the local level. In the same way divisions should undertake the evaluation of systems of care, cost/benefit studies, and medical audit. Community physicians with responsibilities for hospitals within their own areas should promote and actively support such studies. At the present time there is an unfortunate tendency for hospital doctors to regard community physicians as administrators who issue directives but do not wish to become involved in patient care and service improvements. There are faults on both sides and it must be admitted that some community physicians become totally preoccupied with the administrative role; herein lies an urgent problem for the Faculty of Community Medicine; I would again stress the theme of unity within the medical profession and this includes, most importantly, our colleagues in this new Faculty.

The new national consultative machinery could help greatly in the implementation of research results. Let me illustrate the need for its involvement by an example, and then indicate the way in which action might be undertaken successfully. As long ago as 1959 an RCT established the value of oral anticoagulants in the prevention of venous thrombo-embolism in patients who sustain fractures of the femoral neck (15). This provided incontrovertible evidence upon which orthopaedic surgeons could have been expected to plan a prophylactic policy. The extent to which the evidence was acted upon was investigated some sixteen years later by Mitchell (16) who conducted a postal survey throughout the United Kingdom of current practice in the diagnosis and prevention of deep venous thrombosis in elderly patients with hip fractures. A 64 per cent response from over 400 orthopaedic surgeons was received and only 3 per cent routinely prescribed prophylactic anticoagulants. These workers also conducted their own controlled trial and confirmed that benefit rather than harm results from prophylactic anticoagulation in this group of patients. There is clearly no need for yet a further controlled trial but by what method can the incorporation of these findings into routine practice be assured? I do not believe that any health authority today would issue an edict to the effect that prophylactic anticoagulation is mandatory in this group of patients; one can almost picture the rising of professional hackles! And yet this change in management—and several other examples could have been given—should be introduced generally. I suggest that the appropriate specialist sub-committee of the NMCC, consisting as it does of members of the profession, should accept the responsibility of preparing a memorandum for circulation by them to their colleagues. I have raised this course of action at a meeting of the Specialist Sub-committee in General Surgery and was gratified to find that it gained approval.

Implementation of research results will also be facilitated if the local health authority is made aware of the implications of the research at an early stage. Thus if a project on computing in medicine in a hospital is given financial support from a research organization, it is important that the senior medical administrators in that area are aware of its objectives, and are in a position to estimate the continuing support that may be required if the research has a successful outcome.

Finally, increasing specialization has led to the formation of more and more specialist societies and I urge that, where appropriate, societies encourage the introduction of plenary sessions offering general as opposed to specialized research presentations. This has recently been accepted by the Surgical Research Society which has also introduced the concept of presenting review papers which must be given in a form comprehensible to all members, irrespective of special interest.

10

Reflections on personal research with cost implications

New knowledge and new technology in medicine, unlike that in most other industries, tends to result in rising costs rather than in cost saving and yet it can be assumed that new and revolutionary discoveries should, and will, continue to be made. The cost of expanding medical technology is now beginning to receive more attention than in the past, and Hiatt (17) has raised the question as to how much of our resources should be devoted to the development of such sophisticated technologies as the artificial heart: 'proof of effectiveness by itself cannot justify the unlimited spread of new technology. Some technologies will be so costly in relation to benefits that society will be forced to renounce them.' I do not suggest that the quest of new knowledge be abandoned or hindered in any way, but there is clearly a growing need for research which has as its objective cost/effect evaluation of a new technology prior to its general introduction within the health service. In the UK, we have made our share of errors in this regard but some very costly blunders have been avoided. Two examples will suffice.

It has been known for some time that general hypothermia reduces the metabolic demands of most tissues and that it will suspend gastric digestion in most mammals; fish alone provide an exemption. In 1959 Wangensteen and his colleagues (18) achieved local hypothermia of the stomach in dogs and in man by circulating a cold solution through an in-dwelling gastric balloon. These workers then proceeded to study the possibility that the technique could be used to suppress peptic digestion and accelerate healing of stomach ulcers. Alive to the past behaviour of doctors, several industrial companies developed attractive machines capable of producing controlled freezing of the stomach; 2,500 such machines were in use in the USA by the late 1960s. In this country the MRC selected a few clinical academic units (including my surgical unit in the University of Sheffield), supplied the necessary gastric freezing equipment, and supported well-focused experimental and clinical research. As a result the ineffectiveness of freezing as a treatment for peptic ulcer was quickly established and a growing number of hospital demands for expensive freezing machines was properly countered.

Around this time also there was a surge of enthusiasm for the use of hyperbaric oxygen in a number of acute illness situations ranging from surgical infections through carbon monoxide poisoning to acute myocardial infarction—to mention only a few. Hyperbaric installations are not only very expensive to design and produce but they require the constant support of engineering as well as medical and nursing staff, and so the possibility of providing a pressure chamber for all large hospitals had begun to pose a major problem to the health departments. On appointment to the Regius Chair of Surgery in Glasgow University I found myself the curator of the best-equipped pressure chamber in the UK and head of a research group which had already gained a reputation for high quality and relevant scientific work in this field. The MRC, responding to the Health Department problem (a decade before Rothschild) persuaded me of the importance of continuing research in this field and, in particular, of endeavouring to evaluate the place of hyperbaric oxygen therapy in hospital medicine. In brief, the very real possibility that many major hospitals, and all new hospitals, would require to be furnished with a complete hyperbaric installation was avoided. This form of therapy does have a place, but a very limited one, and our final recommendation was that three hyperbaric units strategically placed in the UK, including the Royal Navy installation at Portsmouth, would be adequate provision for the foreseen needs in this country. The work of the Glasgow research team under the guidance of Dr I. McA. Ledingham was essentially of a biomedical nature and important additions to knowledge were made in cardiac, respiratory, and renal physiology some of which have led to a better understanding of the care of the critically ill. In addition, the younger graduate workers in the team changed annually and so a series of young physicians, surgeons, and anaesthetists gained a research training. It can be seen that work in the biomedical field was necessary to achieve an important health service operational research objective and this illustrates the interrelationship of the various branches of medical research.

It is worthy of note that these two examples show that Cochrane's priorities for research in the general applied area were recognized and had been fulfilled, before he had promoted them: withholding the introduction of new drugs and therapeutic procedures unless they are more effective (or equally effective and cheaper) than existing therapies; determining the optimum application of those therapies about which there is any doubt. The very considerable impact of Archie Cochrane's Rock Carling monograph reveals, however, that the medical profession and many medical scientists required his advocacy.

Cochrane has also encouraged us to embark on a very long term evaluation of *all* existing therapies, slowly excluding those shown to be ineffective or too dangerous. If such a programme is to have a chance of being cost-effective it would be essential that results are rigorously implemented. On the basis of past experience my serum hope level is at a dangerously low level!

There is an aspect of controlled trials which tends to be forgotten, namely, that years of careful endeavour (to say nothing of cost) may yield equivocal results. This has been, in large measure, my own experience of trials in the surgical treatment of chronic duodenal ulcer.

The first adequately controlled trial in the surgical management of duodenal ulcer was begun in the Western Infirmary, Glasgow, in 1955. Initially it included three operations: partial gastrectomy, truncal vagotomy with gastrojejunostomy, and gastrojejunostomy alone; at that time it was thought that gastrojejunostomy by itself, a simple and safe operation, might be an acceptable elective operation for duodenal ulcer. However, it took the inclusion of the first sixty patients only in this trial (twenty to each group) to show clearly that gastrojejunostomy by itself carried an unacceptable incidence of recurrent ulcer. From my personal involvement and knowledge of this, and other such trials, this is the one hard fact which emerged and I am relieved to be able to report that, save for a few special indications for its use, gastrojejunostomy has now been eliminated from the repertoire of the ulcer surgeon. This first Glasgow trial continued by allocating further patients to the other two operations and the results in male patients were assessed by Cox (19) (1968) who made the follow-up assessments at comprehensive, standardized interviews. He concluded that insignificant differences existed between the results of partial gastrectomy and truncal vagotomy with gastrojejunostomy.

By 1959, when Goligher and his colleagues initiated a randomized controlled trial (RCT) in the same field, a new operation had gained favour in the USA; antrectomy with truncal vagotomy was promoted on the theoretical ground that it would ablate the two main drives on gastric acid secretion, the nervous drive through the vagus and the hormonal drive from the gastrin secreting antrum of the stomach, thereby reducing acid levels to an extent which should virtually eliminate recurrent ulcer. And so, this operation as well as partial gastrectomy, and truncal vagotomy with gastrojejunostomy was included in what has become recognized as a classic among surgical trials. The detailed results of follow-up through the years have been reported from time to time and the follow-up now extends well beyond a ten-year period. In brief, the over-all clinical grading of results have at all times revealed that approximately the same numbers from each operative group fell into each clinical grade, from the best (no symptoms) to the worst (with symptoms enough to interfere with work or enjoyment of life).

Whatever their faults, surgeons do not lack ingenuity! Since that time new operations have been proposed and it would be fair to say that each has had an acceptable physiological basis. Occasionally the protagonist of a new operation has been so convinced of its outstanding advantages that he failed to initiate early controlled evaluation; however, most academic surgeons no longer require to be persuaded of the need for controlled studies and each new operation has been, or is being, subjected to scrutiny. At this time I have no option but to report that we still do not have a clear leader as the operation of choice in the surgical treatment of duodenal ulcer: one may possess the advantage of a very low immediate mortality rate; another, less satisfactory in this regard, can carry the lowest risk if recurrent ulcer but may at the same time carry a slightly higher incidence of late post-operative sequelae. Fortunately the operations in regular use give acceptably good results in about 90 per cent of patients; the quest of perfection is not easy!

Perhaps because it is inherent in my surgical temperament, I find it difficult to go all the way with Cochrane in his objective 'to evaluate all existing therapies, slowly excluding those shown to be ineffective or too dangerous'; I see this exercise as excessively tedious, too lacking in the stimulation of enthusiasm for those involved, and too costly. We must be selective in deciding therapies that require such arduous evaluation. There are many nostrums still prescribed by doctors which can be rooted out and discarded without the need to apply the rigid scrutiny of RCTs.

Doctors gain a considerable part of their work satisfaction from the act of making a diagnosis; for some, this objective becomes an end in itself. I have no difficulty in recalling that this was my greatest satisfaction when a house physician: the diagnosis of neurological disorders and the intellectual challenge of locating a lesion in the brain or in the spinal cord prevented me, for a time, from the full realization that I was totally incapable of responding to a patient's call for help. The diagnostic aids to which I had recourse could all be employed at the bedside: observation, clinical examination including the use of a pin, a tendon hammer, and a tuning fork, and the occasional resort to lumbar puncture. It was an inexpensive intellectual exercise. Since then, increasingly sophisticated and expensive techniques have become available for the diagnosis of disease and paraclinical empires have grown up in biochemistry, radiology, clinical physics, and the foundations laid for clinical immunology. Cost/effective studies are few and it is of the utmost importance that doctors and medical research workers, with the assistance of interested economists, attack the problem of reducing the number of tests required to reach a diagnosis on which treatment will be based. The present habit of adding a new investigation to the already lengthy list of existing investigations can be upheld only if the results of all, when taken together, improve the accuracy of diagnosis and influence beneficially management and outcome.

The Hospital Health Service Research Unit in the Western Infirmary, Glasgow (supported jointly by the Nuffield Provincial Hospitals Trust and the SHHD) has begun to study this escalating problem. In his contribution to *A Question of Quality* the Honorary Director, Professor Graham Wilson (20), has pointed out that 'despite an increasing amount of available information about patients, diagnosis was not becoming easier as might have been expected. Indeed the situation was even becoming more confused by the multiplicity of tests and some of the investigations used were expensive, possibly hazardous and of uncertain value.' A member of the Unit, Dr Knill-Jones, has shown how the use of statistical techniques and the computation of probabilities can greatly simplify the process of diagnosis in the jaundiced patient, and enhance the accuracy of the conclusion reached from standard tests alone. It has already been demonstrated that the results of the method compare favourably with those of the general physician, that this is achieved using the cheapest and most readily available tests, and that it is applicable in the out-patient clinic. This work is being continued along the lines of developing simple decision trees based on four initial questions and investigations; mathematical ability is not required and these could become important aids to clinical decision-making by the less experienced members of the caring professions. If this can be achieved by the posing of a few critical questions and the use of a few selected diagnostic tests there can be no excuse for subjecting a patient to further investigations, each one of which may increase the patient's anxiety, and will certainly increase the health service bill.

The introduction of a new test should demand clear evidence of its reliability, reproducibility, and diagnostic value. It must then be evaluated against other tests already in practice which have a similar objective. Acceptance of the new test will, in most instances, mean the abandonment of one or more of those already in current practice.

As these are personal reflections I will permit myself the luxury of briefly mentioning a test which I introduced in 1953. Prior to that time a completely satisfactory test of gastric acid secretion was not available. With the advent of the standard antihistamine group of drugs it was considered by us in the Department of

Surgery (Glasgow) that these could be turned to good account in reducing acid secretion which, in turn, is known to be beneficial in the treatment of peptic ulcer. The idea was based on the fact that histamine is generally accepted by physiologists to participate intimately in the production of stomach acid. Suffice it to say that the antihistamines had no beneficial effect on ulcer symptoms and we, among others, showed that this was due to the fact that they did not inhibit the production of gastric acid secretion. I recognized this as a surprising anomaly and even went so far in my thinking to realize that herein might lie the key which could open the door to a successful non-surgical treatment of duodenal ulcer. However, I failed to grasp the big opportunity and selected a lesser one (more of this later). By using an antihistamine to counteract the undesirable generalized effects of an injection of histamine it was found possible to deliver to the stomach a dose of histamine which would maximally stimulate the acid secreting cells. This established a new principle in tests of gastric acid secretion.

Previous tests using such stimulants as caffeine, gruel, and alcohol did not stimulate the stomach maximally and so a different result could occur in one patient on multiple testing; the 'augmented histamine test' had the great benefit of reproducibility. Perhaps for this reason it was quickly accepted for clinical use and its predecessors were abandoned—the desirable sequence of events on the introduction of a new investigation. More recently it became clear that some clinicians were using this test routinely in many patients with dyspepsia even when the diagnosis of peptic ulcer had been made unequivocally by radiological or endoscopic means, and so we decided to study the precise place of the investigation in clinical practice, showed this to be exceedingly limited now that more precise diagnostic tests are available, and published this advice both in the UK and in the USA. In short, the group that advocated the introduction of a test has now advocated its near abandonment save on special indications, and as a clinical research tool. I believe that there is a message here.

11

Future trends in medical research

It is with humility, and considerable trepidation, that I gaze into the crystal ball and dare to predict trends in medical research at the beginning of the twenty-first century. Lacking the depth of knowledge required to cover the entire field of research in medicine I must be selective and, before treading the relatively unfamiliar paths of prenatal diagnosis, screening procedures, pharmacology, molecular genetics and genetic engineering, environmental pollution, and epidemiological research, I will begin with what is for me the more familiar surgical arena. However, even here, I am chastened by the recollection that few predictions have proved so wrong as that made by a famous surgeon, prior to the discovery of anaesthesia and infection, to the effect that surgery had reached its peak and could not be expected to make any further progress! Since then the abdomen, the thorax, and the skull have yielded in turn to the surgeon's knife—to say nothing of organ transplantation. And yet, how could he have anticipated the revolution which followed the discovery of anaesthesia and the development, some twenty years later, of the antiseptic method by Joseph Lister? It has become customary to divide the history of surgery into two epochs—before Lister and after Lister—and there is an inference that sepsis is no longer with us. This is far from true and some data from the United States are of interest: in a total of 18·8 million surgical procedures there were 1·4 million infections. The cost in treatment, stay in hospital, and loss of income was estimated to be approximately $9 billion per annum. This must be an area for continued basic, clinical, and health services research with the combined objective of effectively lowering the risk and frequency of surgical infection.

The remarkable development of surgery in the post-Listerian era has oft been told, but it is salutary to consider briefly the continuous struggle which has taken place since then against pathogenic bacteria. Lister's approach was an offensive one in that he used *antiseptics* which destroyed not only bacteria but had damaging effects on healthy tissues. But the next phase in the struggle proved to be even more successful, namely, the pacifist or defensive approach: *asepsis* left the defences of the body intact, did not destroy healthy tissues, and quickly proved its superiority. Following the introduction of antibiotics, surgeons tried the preventive approach, and used these new agents as prophylactics, but we have now learned that the resistance of bacteria increased and there developed resistant strains which, in the last analysis, left the balance of power unchanged. We are now learning to keep the antibiotic weapon in reserve for major bacterial invasions when they are likely to be more effective in their encounter with non-resistant bacteria. We have now reached a stage akin to stalemate in war: new antibiotic weapons are being developed by the pharmaceutical industries but these in turn lose effectiveness as bacteria develop resistance; as a result we have a continuing arms race and research in this area is mandatory.

Of course progress has been made in the prevention of infection in clean surgical operations but even here the incidence of wound infection varies from 1 to 10 per cent and causes appreciable morbidity. In critically ill or severely injured patients sepsis remains the major factor in determining a fatal outcome. Today the greatest threat comes from the gram negative group of organisms which now predominate in our hospitals.

It must be concluded that there is a continuing need for research in the broad area of microbial infections and, more particularly, in relation to hospital surgical practice.

RESEARCH WILL DIMINISH THE NEED FOR SURGICAL TREATMENT

All surgeons enjoy the craft of surgery but some, in addition, have as a firm objective the desirability of reducing the need for surgical intervention. There are some areas, at present within the surgical province, that can be expected to be eliminated by future research.

Endocrine surgery is one such area. Some twenty years ago the advent of the anti-thyroid drugs seemed to herald the abandonment of thyroidectomy in the treatment of hyperthyroidism; although this has not yet come to pass the operation is much less common today and further research in this area can be expected to eliminate the need for surgery altogether. Again, those of us with a special interest in the surgery of the adrenal gland find our surgical practice diminishing: already, pharmacological research has led to the development of antagonists to each of the hormones secreted by the adrenal and more and more patients are restored to health without the risks, slight though these are, of surgical intervention. It is not difficult to envisage that progress will be made along similar lines in the management of hyperinsulinism and hyperparathyroidism.

Surgeons may, however, find a role in the management of diabetes. Although the discovery and use of insulin has led to the control of the diabetic patient's blood sugar problems and thus allowed him to lead a near-normal life, insulin does not prevent the effects of diabetes on the blood vessels and affected patients are prone to early death from atherosclerosis as it hits the cerebral vessels, producing strokes, and the vessels of the heart, producing myocardial infarction. Further research into the problems of organ rejection together with continuing improvement in microsurgical techniques may permit safe transplantation of the entire pancreas, and the resultant production of endogenous insulin *may* prevent the onset of these hazards. Alternatively, a successful outcome to current research aimed at the culture of islet cells of the pancreas (insulin-producing cells) may permit their injection into an appropriate organ such as the spleen where they can survive and produce the diabetic patient's proper and natural insulin requirements. This technique, by avoiding major transplantation surgery, has great potential. It is not beyond the bounds of probability that other deficiency states will respond to similar approaches.

Reference has been made earlier to the advent of new drugs which have a profound effect on controlling acid secretionby the stomach and further research in this area may lead to non-surgical treatment for many of the thousands of patients with duodenal ulcer. The story of recent events merits telling.

In the late 1960s James Black (22) re-examined the anomaly whereby standard antihistamines fail to antagonize the action of histamine and developed the hypothesis that there must be at least two types of histamine receptor: the H1 receptor was regarded as being responsible for the majority of the actions of histamine throughout the body; the H2 receptor was postulated to relate to the acid secreting cell of the stomach and, unlike H1 receptors, would not be blocked by conventional antihistaminics. The story is a fascinating one but suffice it to say that a search was then introduced for an H2 receptor antagonist, and this was rewarded by success in the course of a few years. The first active drug to be used in man was metiamide which was shown to be a potent inhibitor of the secretion of acid by the stomach cells and capable of inducing rapid healing of even the most fulminating forms of peptic ulcer. However, while it was still being studied by selected clinical investigators, a few patients were found to develop a fall in the white blood cell count to an extent which made them susceptible to fulminating infection. A similar side-effect had occurred with the earliest of the thiourea drugs used in the treatment of hyperthyroidism and, acting on previous experience, the chemists proceeded to exclude the sulphur radicle from the chemical structure of metiamide. This has led to the introduction cimetidine which has been shown to be equally effective in controlling gastric acid and is apparently free from the undesired side effect of its predecessor. The very early results of limited RCTs are now becoming available and it must be said that these are encouraging but, before a thorough evaluation had been completed, the flood-gates for the indiscriminate use of this potentially valuable agent have been opened. Its general availability was commented upon recently by the mass media, sufferers from dyspepsia can be expected to demand the new wonder drug, benefit is being assumed without serious consideration of cost, and all this will take place while important questions remain to be answered. Will the patient require to stay on permanent cimetidine treatment, like the diabetic on insulin? Will there be a rebound phenomenon, perhaps leading to ulcer complications, if and when the patient stops treatment? Will side-effects, hitherto unsuspected, become apparent with continued usage? Will long-term cimetidine therapy give better over-all results than modern surgical treatment—which has recently been shown to give almost 90 per cent of good results as assessed by a computer-based trial recently completed by the University Department of Surgery, Western Infirmary, Glasgow? The time is ripe for a controlled trial of standard surgical treatment for duodenal ulcer against long-term treatment with cimetidine. Trials of this sort should be concerned not only with an assessment of the long-term clinical result but with the relative costs of the two forms of treatment. It could be that an operation which offers a 90 per cent chance of a good result, carries a very low mortality, and does not require the patient to continue taking tablets for the rest of his life is preferable to long-term drug therapy. We need to know the answer to such questions.

The present heavy load of cardiovascular surgery reflects the growing health problem of intermittent claudication, strokes, and ischaemic heart disease. Although large sums of money are being spent on research related to atherosclerosis there has so far been little practical impact. At the present time emphasis is being placed on preventive measures such as no smoking, dietary change with reduced lipid ingestion, and the taking of adequate exercise. For each of these there is evidence, but do we seriously believe that a healthy individual will act on evidence which is far from 'hard' particularly when he does not wish to give up anything unless he is certain that he himself will benefit? As Professor Dunphy has said, 'I suspect that if we could find evidence that roast beef properly cooked and served with roast potatoes and Yorkshire pudding was a principal factor, the dietary habits in the United States and Great Britain would change very little'. Behavioural change is maybe the next great challenge but it will take time. Concurrently, research must continue into the fundamental understanding of the pathophysiology of arterial disease and success here would result in a major diminution in surgical requirement. Again, increasingly sophisticated diagnostic techniques will undoubtedly detect atherosclerotic changes at a very early stage which could respond to medication or to the infusion of solutions (not yet developed) into the affected vessels. While I suspect that few cardiac surgeons would agree with me, I am optimistic that research on ischaemic heart disease will lead to a falling requirement for coronary artery surgery by the beginning of the twenty-first century.

John Charnley has pioneered hip joint replacement and an ageing population will put a growing demand on this type of surgery. However, hopefully, research directed towards our fuller understanding of rheumatoid arthritis may well diminish the need for surgical replacement of the smaller joints.

My colleagues in urological surgery are already recording a rising demand for prostatectomy—scarcely surprising as more and more men live longer. Research is urgently required towards a non-surgical treatment for prostatism; and if this problem is not solved by the end of the century the logistics of the surgical demand will be staggering.

One can with some certainty predict that major injuries will continue to make increasing demands on the surgeon. Accidents and trauma have already been identified by the health departments and by the MRC as priority research areas and it is essential that all the relevant disciplines of medical research be involved without delay. Epidemiological studies are clearly required. Significant advances are being made in the management of critically ill or injured patients; we are already beginning to see recovery, with good quality of life, from near-lethal injuries and progress in this direction is certain to continue. There is still room for improvement in respiratory and circulatory support systems and further research is likely to be productive. It is here that computers will find one of their major uses. They are already used to register input data concerning pulse rate, respiration, temperature, blood gases, etc., together with signalling when these data deviate from normal values. However, the apparatus will reach a stage when it can be programmed for active use in treatment; thus it is likely to be able to control the automatic regulation of blood transfusion, fluid and electrolyte administration, and even for providing the information which will help to decide whether further surgery is, or is not, indicated. The full potential of computers applied to medicine is still to be realized and it is likely that there will be further major developments in the diagnostic field, in treatment, and in the recording and evaluation of all patient data both for clinical and for research purposes.

A modicum of confidence gained by considering research trends in surgery, I will now turn attention to other selected areas.

PRENATAL DIAGNOSIS AND SELECTIVE ABORTION

This subject has been discussed in detail and with typical clarity by Professor Harry Harris (23) in his 1974 Rock Carling monograph. Further research in this area, followed by careful and discriminating implementation of the results, should undoubtedly lead to a major and beneficial advance in medicine by the beginning of the next century. Important basic information is already available. Thus it is estimated that about 15 per cent of recognized pregnancies end in the first trimester by spontaneous abortion and that 50 per cent of such abortions have some chromosomal aberration; 10 per cent have neural tube defects. The purpose of prenatal screening will be to identify in the second trimester those abnormal foetuses which survive beyond the first three months.

We are therefore able to focus on the use of diagnostic techniques at about 16 weeks gestation. The technique of withdrawal of amniotic fluid is already well established and, in addition, the development of fibre-optic instruments allows the inspection of the foetus and withdrawal of blood from a superficial vein for special study. Another recent advance which offers hope of extending the screening process is the demonstration of raised blood α foetoprotein levels in a proportion of pregnancies with a neural tube defect between 12 and 22 weeks; the level falls as pregnancy advances and the test becomes valueless in the later stages of pregnancy. Although occasional false negative results are obtained, the sensitivity of the test has reached the stage when a 100 per cent pick-up rate has been recorded for anencephaly and between 75 and 80 per cent for spina bifeds in centres at Edinburgh, Glasgow, and Belfast (Ferguson-Smith, 1976 [24]). It can be predicted that within the next few years the results will be sufficiently encouraging to take research further and evaluate the results of prenatal screening in the community.

At the present time the most highly developed branch of the subject is that concerned with chromosomal abnormalities and it may be that it is in relation to the prenatal diagnosis of metabolic and other non-chromosomal defects that the main thrust of new research and development can be anticipated. It is worth emphasizing that there are some inherited diseases, of particular importance because of their high incidence and considerable morbidity, which will eventually be capable of prenatal diagnosis. These include cystic fibrosis and the various forms of thalassaemia. Even now important advances have been made in relation to these conditions but it is already apparent that the services required could at this time be made available only in a few highly developed countries; unfortunately the incidence of the diseases mentioned is greatest in underdeveloped countries in which the prevention and treatment of other forms of illness merit higher priority. However, as Harris has pointed out, even in more advanced countries with established health services, the introduction of prenatal diagnosis for conditions such as B-thalassaemia would raise formidable problems:

> Even in England where the number of people who have come, or whose ancestors came, from parts of the world with high frequencies of these genes is proportionally very much less, the actual number of pregnancies 'at risk' are quite appreciable. An illustration of this problem as it occurs in a particular community is provided by the results of a study of the Cypriot population in three boroughs of north London, which suggested that about 1 in 7 are heterozygous for a B-thalassaemia gene, and that about 0·5% of the new-born may be expected to suffer from B-thalassaemia major.

So far I have been discussing 'negative' eugenics in which the policy is aimed at preventing the birth of those who are considered to harbour undesirable genes so that poor-quality lives can be avoided and so that there may be a reduced incidence of the abnormality in subsequent generations. Harris has emphasized the dangers of accepting 'positive' eugenics as a public policy since this would have the objective of increasing the incidence of genes thought to result in desirable human qualities. The obvious threat of such a policy would be the possibility that it would encourage totalitarian governments to create a race of individuals who could be used to maintain power. This aspect of eugenics tends to emerge in debates on the ethics of selective abortion but it is important to emphasize the real benefits that the procedure could confer if confined to 'negative' eugenics. To be able to offer to parents, who have already had an abnormal child, the opportunity of being confident that the next pregnancy would result in a normal infant is surely a considerable achievement. I judge that the results of continuing research in this area will in due course have long-term individual and social acceptability and benefit.

EVALUATION OF SCREENING PROCEDURES

One of the earliest records of a screening procedure relates to the papal state of Avignon where Queen Jane I set up a 'publick brothel' in 1347. This required the provision of weekly examination of the staff by the abbess and a surgeon. There is no record of the sensitivity or specificity of the examinations employed, or of the inter-observer error between the abbess and the surgeon, but there can be little doubt that, like most subsequent screening procedures it was established because it seemed a good idea rather than that it had been shown to be of proven worth. Even today we have no grounds for complacency and it is now a matter of importance to make every attempt to measure the outcome in a group offered screening, and to compare this with the outcome of a control group not offered screening. It is by this method alone that we can determine whether our good intentions have in fact been fulfilled, and it must be admitted that there are very few areas in which this has been demonstrated.

Screening methods have been advocated and introduced at all ages.

Screening at-risk relatives of congenitally abnormal children in order to give them genetic counselling has been practised for some time. While few would doubt the wisdom of offering advice, while leaving the individual to make his or her own decision, there is no hard evidence of its beneficial effect.

Antenatal screening has been established for many years and there is good evidence here for the worth of some of its procedures, and others await evaluation. The detection of Rhesus negativity in the mother and then administering anti-D immunoglobulin has virtually eliminated the need for exchange transfusion in Rhesus incompatibility. The detection of severe gestational diabetes has also been proven of value in reducing the risks to the foetus.

In the neonatal period screening for phenylketonuria has unquestionably proved its worth. There is a highly significant difference in intelligence levels and social independence between two comparable groups of affected patients, one treated early as a result of screening and the other untreated, or treated late. The value of other procedures carried out on the newborn remains uncertain, for example detection of dislocation of the hip and congenital heart disease have been introduced without adequate evaluation so that it is now almost impossible to judge their worth.

Of the vast array of screening procedures advocated during infancy and childhood, remarkably few have been adequately evaluated and even the two most hopeful areas of infant screening, searching for hearing and squint defects, have yet to be substantiated as of real benefit. Furthermore, the response rate of those most in need is unknown.

In the adult, comprehensive screening is now only established on a UK basis for antenatal services and for cervical cytology. It is significant that after almost twenty years we still are unable to determine if the latter leads to real benefit.

Geriatric screening is a virtually unexplored field for research and one in which it may be worthwhile applying screening with different objectives, namely, care. It is mandatory that, prior to the introduction of screening, the evaluation is planned to demonstrate which tests are of value and what services can be mobilized.

The present status of our screening services is that they are supported more by enthusiasm and rhetoric than by carefully assembled scientific information and research continues to be needed in this field. An effective treatment should be available before screening programmes are mounted. The question of cost effectiveness is exceedingly complex and many factors merit comparison: the cost of testing compared with conventional diagnostic costs; the cost of diagnosis, including all false positives; treatment costs; the cost in time taken over the screening procedures; 'imponderable costs' such as inconvenience and the psychological disturbance engendered in a proportion of the screened population. And the difficulty does not stop here. Even if evaluation demonstrates the worth of screening there is the problem of obtaining high compliance rates and the method of approach may require to be adapted to suit the cultural pattern of differing social groups.

To conclude on an optimistic note, the earliest and highly successful screening for pulmonary tuberculosis by mass radiography included in its outcome four separate activities. It provided a means of identifying quiescent disease and so prevented an individual from progression to advanced disease as well as preventing him from continuing to be a source of infection to members of his nearby community; it offered hope of cure for the individual affected by the disease; it identified individuals with disability beyond the bounds of cure but nevertheless in need of care; it provided some administrative information to the health services so that they were able to plan more economically. These four functions—prevention, cure, care, and administration—may through future research be fulfilled in a growing number of screening procedures.

THE FUTURE OF PHARMACOLOGICAL RESEARCH

Pharmacological research has developed very rapidly in the course of the last twenty or thirty years. This has been due in no small measure to the research efforts of the pharmaceutical industry in the areas of chemical synthesis, mechanism of drug action, and toxicology. This industrial drive has been supplemented by university research, and continuation of profitable collaboration is to be encouraged. It is unlikely, however, that the public's growing demand for drugs which will cure, have a total absence of side-effects, and be inexpensive will be fulfilled. This demand is at odds with the recurring public cry against the use of animals for pharmacological research which, if followed, would reduce the present scrutiny given to possible toxic action. An alternative is to restrict the animal testing stage to what is absolutely necessary and to introduce more quickly (but with reasonable precautions) clinical testing. If the issue were to be forced, it is doubtful if public opinion would regard this as an acceptable alternative.

Research is likely to be along two different lines. Firstly, there will be a continuation of the systematic approach in which there is scanning of a vast number of potential new products. In this method the acute observer may occasionally note an unexpected action which can give a new lead but this form of research activity is both tedious and expensive. Secondly, the few exciting new drugs which we will almost certainly see by the turn of the century, are likely to be the result of advances in fundamental biology: knowledge gained at this level points the way to new therapeutic attacks. This has already been illustrated in relation to the new concept of the existence of at least two types of histamine receptor within the body which led to the synthesis of compounds which have considerable potential in the non-surgical treatment of peptic ulceration. A time can be envisaged when we will know sufficient about the metabolism of lipids to commence a search for effective drug therapy in atherosclerosis. Again, while some progress has been made, our knowledge of the basic metabolic processes within the nervous system can be expected to grow to the point at which we will have greater control over a growing number of mental and behavioural disturbances.

Finally, observation and research on drug interaction must continue. The prescribing habits of many doctors leave much to be desired and it has to be admitted that not a few patients are advised to take more than a few drugs at any one time. It would be comforting, but incorrect, to think that the possible interactions among these drugs was known by the prescriber admittedly, in many instances, because the knowledge is not available. This situation has led to the need for more clinical pharmacologists and the demand for such trained personnel will increase. It may be that the cost to the NHS of an adequate number of clinical pharmacologists will be offset by their influence on the prescribing habits of their clinical colleagues and by improvements in the quality of care.

MOLECULAR BIOLOGY WITH SPECIAL REFERENCE TO MOLECULAR GENETICS

Molecular biology is a wide subject covering studies of the function and structure of enzymes, the constitution and operation of cell membranes, molecular genetics, and so on. New, unexpected, and exciting facts emerge with startling rapidity and additions to fundamental knowledge have been truly immense. Failing to comprehend the complexities of this branch of science, clinicians have tended to become disenchanted and to ask when the 'pay off' can be anticipated.

Selecting molecular genetics for special consideration, it should be remembered that it is just twenty years ago since Crick and Watson advanced their hypothesis of the double helical structure of DNA. Few would disagree that their concept has not been surpassed by any other idea in the long story of scientific endeavour. The last two decades has seen molecular genetics provide the framework for our growing understanding of how living systems work and how they may change with time. Although viruses and bacteria provide the usual experimental model for the molecular geneticist, the knowledge gained is now being applied to higher organisms and it can be anticipated that the potential of this scientific discipline will be fulfilled in terms of practical application by the turn of the century. First, the vast range of different types of virus is now gradually being revealed and this will lead to a better understanding of virus diseases in man and, in due course, to the treatment or even prevention of some of them. Secondly, viral agents have been identified which can transform eukaryotic cells into cancerous forms, and this has become one of the most active areas of cancer research at the present time. Some experts believe that this approach will lead to a resolution of the cancer problem. Thirdly, and I quote C. H. Waddington (25): 'Molecular genetics holds out the hope of a new and potentially extremely powerful method of analysing one of the great problems of biology in which our understanding is, as yet, perhaps most backward of all, namely the correlation of nervous activities underlying the phenomena of co-ordinated behaviour, and eventually of "mind".' Brenner and his colleagues (26) are studying this challenging problem using a small nematode worm (*C. elegans*), exploring the genetic properties of this organism and developing methods planned to provide a complete and detailed structure of its nervous system. 'Tracing the connections between genes and behaviour is a fascinating but very difficult problem. One is aware of the possibility that understanding of this might well involve solving all the outstanding questions of biology.' It seems very unlikely that this century will see the dawn of that great day but the forecast of a scientist as knowledgeable as Brenner is worthy of respect. It is difficult at this time to contemplate the benefits which could accrue to mankind; meantime, let us recognize the past and current achievements of fundamental science and the importance of its continued, adequate support.

Public interest has been aroused in the past two or three years concerning 'genetic engineering', a technique by which genetic material can be passed from one organism to another.

In July 1974 the Advisory Board to the Research Councils agreed to establish a working party under the chairmanship of Lord Ashby with the following terms of reference: 'To assess the potential benefits and potential hazards of techniques which allow the experimental manipulation of the genetic composition of micro-organisms; and to report to the ABRC.' The problems to be assessed had already received considerable publicity in the press and through the mass media and, as they were causing both interest and concern outwith the scientific community, the working party wisely decided that it was in the public interest to report their assessment in such a way that it would be intelligible to people unfamiliar with the language of modern genetics. The success with which this intention was met can be judged by the fact that I consider that I am capable of making a brief comment on this exciting new area of biological research. I acknowledge here that much of the information used in my commentary comes directly from the *Report of the Working Party on the Experimental Manipulation of the Genetic Composition of Micro-organisms* (Cmnd 5880) (27).

What are the basic facts about this new technique? Those who share my interest in gardening will be well aware that a growing number of F^1 hybrid plants and vegetables are now available. The process of cross-breeding closely related plants (or animals) is an established way of producing new combinations of genetic information. This can also be done experimentally by ionizing radiation or by appropriate chemical treatment. The frequency with which I now select F^1 hybrid seeds is, in a very small way, an indication that some of the induced changes have resulted in highly successful strains. Translated to world needs, we are acquiring the ability to increase the yield and quality of those crops which provide us with our daily food. It should not be forgotten that, in nature, unselective gene recombination is taking place all the time.

Until recently it has not been possible to make a transfer of single genes, or small groups of genes, between unrelated higher organisms. As stated in the Report: 'Now, there are new techniques which hold out promise that new combinations of genetic information may be made, by splicing segments of severed chromosomes together with much greater precision and speed, and in ways which transcend the barriers between unlike organisms.' These techniques have been well described by Ziff (28) in 1973. All that need be said here is that a special enzyme (the restriction enzyme) will cut the DNA threads (chromosomes) of an organism in such a way that segments can unite with other similarly cut DNA segments and become incorporated into the genetic constitution of unlike organisms.

Among other novel techniques is the fusion of cells to form hybrids in ways which bypass the normal sexual process and the subsequent growth in culture of cells containing nuclei from various sources. The working party did not discount the possibility of unpredictable hazards in such experiments and expressed the view that the progress of this kind of work should be monitored with the greatest care by the scientific community.

The potential benefits from the experimental manipulation of genes must be largely speculative at the present time, but in the view of experts in this field of science these are likely to be impressive. The new techniques will increase our understanding of the mechanism of gene action: thus every living animal cell possesses a set of genes but not all of these are active, the expression of some being prevented; transfer of small groups of genes out of their normal environment into bacteria is likely to facilitate the study of how they work and of how they are controlled. This in turn, as mentioned earlier, could lead to an appreciation of how genes cause or permit the development of cancers. Again, segments of DNA could be introduced into *E. coli* where they would multiply as the organism undergoes division and so produce increasing amounts of the selected segments; these in turn could be dissected and their precise function determined. A possible and important practical application would, for example, be the use of the genes responsible for the chemical synthesis of hormones or antibodies, etc.; this envisages bacterial cultures acting as factories for the production of these valuable therapeutic agents. Reference has already been made to the improvement in various crops already achieved by using the relatively inaccurate method of treating genes chemically or by ionizing radiation; the newer techniques should have the advantage of greater precision and could provide a solution to the growing world food shortage. Finally, these techniques have already improved our understanding of bacterial virulence and drug resistance, and further advances in this area can be anticipated.

That potential hazards must be borne in mind was brought clearly into focus in July 1974 when the National Academy of Sciencies of the USA endorsed a statement by the Committee chaired by Professor Paul Berg calling for a temporary halt on certain types of genetic research in order to give time to acquire a clearer assessment of risk. The Academy called for a voluntary world-wide moratorium on the designated research areas, which included those that could result in significant extension of knowledge on drug-resistance in bacteria. This was the stimulus to the setting up of Lord Ashby's working party. It should be emphasized that we have already gained considerable experience of procedures involving the safe handling of dangerous pathogenic organisms and this experience will be helpful in preparing a code of practice. The strategy which has been developed over the years for the safe conduct of hazardous procedures in the study of infectious disease and in the production of some vaccines has been highly successful and the immediate setting up of a Committee of Enquiry into the smallpox outbreak in London in March and April 1973 illustrates the extreme rarity of failure of containment. There are good grounds for public reassurance.

Lord Ashby's working party came to the conclusion that the potential benefits of genetic manipulation by these new techniques are likely to be great and that, subject to rigorous safeguards, research should be allowed to continue.

ENVIRONMENTAL RESEARCH

There will be, and indeed there must be, an adequate programme of research concerned with chemical hazards in our environment. The growing concern of society on the possible dangers of environmental pollution suggests that this is a new phenomenon, but there can be little doubt that conditions in European cities three centuries ago were much worse than we experience today: major epidemics were rife and I suspect that the environment of Western man was more dangerous then, than now.

Man has always lived in a changing world but it is perhaps true to say that the rate of change has accelerated with the technicological revolution and so, whereas society in former times was able to absorb and adapt to it, society today lags in adaptation. This may explain the emotion evoked by mention of the possible risks of chemical, nuclear, and other forms of pollution. Let us not forget, however, that some technicological advances have in themselves done much to improve our environment. Collaboration between several scientific disciplines will be required to meet future research needs.

Formerly, toxicology was concerned mainly with the acute effects of poisonous agents, and these were able to be studied with relative ease in the experimental laboratory. Today, however, there is a growing concern about the possibly deleterious effects of minute amounts of toxic substances in different articles of our diet acting over a prolonged period of time. Chronic studies are required, but the life-span of most experimental animals does not compare with that of man and, in any event, results from animal studies cannot always be translated directly to the human subject. A growing world population also compounds the difficulties. Do we decide to allow a proportion of human beings to die of starvation, or do we increase the yield of crops to keep all alive with the help of sophisticated but potentially hazardous chemical adjuvants? Society's elected representatives must bear the responsibility of facing this dilemma and of providing the answer; the role of the scientist is to conduct any necessary studies, produce the facts and interpret them in a completely objective manner, indicating wherever required any doubts or uncertainties that he may have.

Epidemiology (which will be considered in its broader aspects hereafter) has had major successes in the control of infections and should now be applied increasingly to problems related to chemicals in our food and in our environment. Higgins (29) has demonstrated that epidemiological study of acute outbreaks of poisoning may identify the influence of certain toxic substances in the environment particularly when there is a combination of a specialized industrial activity together with a lack of care in preventing the release of the material in question into the surroundings. It is highly probable that there are many other instances where the suspected agent is dispersed more widely; here, epidemiological studies may at best indicate several possibilities. The uneven distribution of certain types of cancer in various parts of the world is illustrative and this may be due to a varying incidence of as yet unknown environmental factors. Information is lacking and it is evident that scientists will require to use epidemiological methods increasingly, in addition to the traditional scientific disciplines employed in the study of pollution. The need for collaboration has been clearly indicated by Neuberger (30):

> the comprehensive investigation of the possible toxic effect of a particular agent may involve knowledge of the enzymic processes which may be relevant, an understanding of the biology of the cell, an analysis of the movement of the suspected agent between different body compartments, and a knowledge of the industrial process involved. In order to analyse the problem fully, the scientist may have to use methods of epidemiology as well as a variety of other scientific disciplines. This great variety of scientific approaches makes the whole field difficult to organise, but at the same time the diversity of techniques represents an important challenge to the scientist who wishes to use his skill in the pursuit of social ends.

EPIDEMIOLOGY

The careful observation and recording of what happens to man in the course of his ordinary life, with particular reference to disease, will make an increasing contribution to medical progress. This scientific approach to the study of disease has the immediate advantage that positive results are directly relevant to man. Again, the opportunity to study large numbers of individuals increases the chance of detecting quite small effects. Those who would detract from the value of the epidemiological method point out that observation alone cannot *prove* that any particular agent is the cause of disease in man. However, as Professor Sir Richard Doll (31) stresses, no amount of argument about observational data can distinguish cause and effect from an unimportant secondary association and, sooner or later, we will require to experiment, modify the human environment, and see what happens: 'if we can do this in a properly controlled way, with random allocation, as was done by fluoridating the water in three out of six towns, or by substituting polyunsaturated for normal fat in the diet, so much the better'. It must be admitted that such studies will be costly in terms of time, effort and money and will require the collaboration of individuals who may even wish to be assured that the modification will prove to be successful—before the study has been undertaken!

Epidemiology, which had its origins in the study of epidemics of infectious disease, has continued to extend its boundaries; with the interested assistance of clinicians it has led to the prevention of a variety of occupational diseases and to the recognition and treatment of several vitamin and nutritional deficiencies; and now, in our time, it is being recognized that the epidemiologist has much to offer preventive medicine across the five continents. While we can scarcely hope for many dramatic advances such as Denis Burkitt's brilliant work on the lymphoma which bears his name, a vast amount of new information can come from defining and characterizing the areas in which a disease is either very common or exceedingly rare. Epidemiological developments of this sort provide opportunities for focused experimental and clinical research. This is well exemplified by an area which is of special interest to members of my own surgical laboratories, namely, carcinoma of the colon. Professor Sir Robert Williams and his colleagues took the opportunity to test the idea that the occurrence of cancer of the colon might be related to the bacterial flora within the bowel. Specimens of stool were collected from healthy adults in high incidence areas (USA and the UK) and low incidence areas (Uganda, India, and Japan). Although the same broad groups of bacteria were present in all, specimens from high incidence areas showed greater numbers of anaerobic bacteroides capable of degrading bile salts by dehydrogenation; there was a close correlation between the incidence of colon cancer and the amount of dihydroxycholanic acids in the faeces—some of which may well be precursors of carcinogens, if indeed they are not carcinogenic themselves. These results have now been extended by the collection of data from other areas and preliminary findings, reported by Sir Richard Doll, indicate that the same relationship holds for affected and unaffected individuals in a particular area. This suggests that a study of the faecal flora could possibly be of value as a predictor of the risk of an individual developing this form of cancer; it also raises the hope that a planned change in intestinal flora, for example by dietary intervention, may diminish the risk. A clue to appropriate dietary intervention may rest in Burkitt's further epidemiological studies on dietary fibre. He has shown that in countries with a low incidence of cancer of the colon the diet contains a great deal of fibre which tends to produce a regular and easy bowel action; in 'more civilized' countries the fibre content of the diet is low, constipation and straining at stool are common, and the incidence of cancer of the colon is significantly higher.

It can be predicted with some confidence that epidemiological studies of this sort can be applied with benefit to a wide variety of conditions including other cancers, coronary artery disease, and multiple sclerosis. While some of the striking variations in incidence will be related to genetic differences, it is likely that most will be shown to be of environmental or behavioural origin. Doll (32) has pointed out: 'sometimes an explanation is thrust on our notice by some accompanying peculiarity of geography or culture; but more often we have to await the impact of a seminal idea like those propounded by Williams and by Burkitt'. The way ahead having been given by epidemiological work, basic or clinical research experiments can be planned.

Epidemiology has also much to offer in the detection of adverse reactions to drugs. Although the procedures developed by the Committee on Safety of Medicines have done much to ensure that a new drug will offer significant benefits and carry a very small risk of harmful effects, it must be admitted that much depends on a doctor's acuity, his sense of suspicion, and his willingness to report in detail. There is a need to develop in this country a system of intensive monitoring along the lines of that developed by Jick and his colleagues in Boston with whom Lawson in Glasgow is now actively collaborating. The feature of this system is that the occurrence of all significant medical events related to the use of a drug are recorded and analysed automatically; it is therefore particularly applicable to hospital practice. It will also be important to organize a system whereby prescriptions can be recorded and linked with an individual's present and subsequent clinical history.

The epidemiologist will also have much to offer in the future in the assessment of need of medical services, and in the evaluation of the services provided to meet that need. This is a matter which has been explored by the Department of Community Medicine in the University of Manchester and it is important that others follow this initiative.

While there should be little disagreement about the desirability for growth in epidemiological research as applied to medicine, there must be concern about the availability of adequately trained research workers in this discipline. The United Kingdom, largely through the work of Bradford Hill and Richard Doll, led the world in epidemiological research but while the USA has built on their pioneering efforts and has produced a growing cadre of epidemiologists, the disciples here have been disappointingly few in number. Applicants for financial support in health services research frequently request the assistance of an epidemiologist and the need for this form of support will often be accepted by the awarding scientific committee; all too often there is great difficulty in finding an adequately trained worker to fill the post. There is therefore an urgent need to encourage the training of professional epidemiological research workers who find problems in this displine challenging and rewarding, and I suggest that this can best be done in the following ways. First, the time has come to support the establishment of more strong departments of community medicine within our medical schools and to ensure that adequate opportunity is given for participation in the teaching of undergraduate students. This view was expressed in the Report of the Royal Commission on Medical Education (7) on general professional training (para. 74):

> there are many branches of clinical medicine in which a greater than average knowledge of community medicine is desirable; opportunities should be created for interested young clinicians in all specialties to get experience in epidemiological research methods, training in epidemiological and statistical aspects of their own specialties, and a simple introduction, in courses provided by

universities, to the principles of management and operational research. Consideration should be given to providing, in all large hospitals, formal instruction in this subject . . .

Secondly, as has been considered elsewhere, the Faculty of Community Medicine must urgently insist that Fellows and Members should become more interested in the study of populations than in attendance at the innumerable committees which have mushroomed since reorganization of the NHS. Thirdly, there is evidence that a growing number of clinical scientists are interested in the research leads which are the product of epidemiological studies: while much could and will emerge from closer collaboration, there is no reason why the clinician should not regard training in epidemiology of at least equal importance to a training in experimental or clinical research techniques. I do not infer that all should have this training but, reverting to my underlying theme, a balance in medical research calls for a balance in the expertise offered by the country's research manpower; those that opt for epidemiological training should be encouraged to do so.

12

An overview of the future

Health is now one of the major industries in this country with a major investment of public funds. This being so, it is a matter for concern that there is so little analytical information about the enterprise. There is little in the way of a health policy as that term is used for other major public industries, and real policy planning is still in its infancy. At the same time there is growing concern at rising costs and gathering doubt that we are getting value for money. Because society had come to believe that medical research would solve all its health problems, and do so speedily, there is a loss of confidence in the value and effectiveness of science and a resultant diminution in the support for the medical sciences. The criticism of our health care system has become incessant so that we are in danger of failing to remember our genuine assets and, more importantly, of failing to be ready to take advantage of the opportunities of medical science which, in the long history of medicine, have never been so promising. An optimist, but I hope not without realism, I believe that in the not very distant future there is the real possibility that man can be rid of the major diseases which now cause concern; if this hope is to be realized, now is the time to overthrow depression about medical science and plan for its bright long-term future.

Although it is unfashionable to say that things have improved greatly over the past fifty years, this is undoubtedly true and we should not overlook the past in our efforts to gain something better for the future; the past informs us of methods for further improvement. McKeown (33), my immediate predecessor as Rock Carling Fellow, has traced the changes in the pattern of mortality in Britain and has shown that expectation of life has increased markedly since death certification began in 1938. I would agree that decreasing mortality from infectious disease played a major part and that much of the decrease occurred before the development of antibiotics and modern medical techniques; McKeown is correct in saying that nutrition, hygiene, and altered behavioural habits take much credit but I cannot accept that the application of the results of medical research have had little effect on mortality and morbidity. When I was a medical student we had a special ward for erysipelas; as a house doctor in the Royal Hospital for Sick Children I spun down the cerebrospinal fluid of infants in the small hours of the morning and when I saw the formation of a 'spider web' I knew that death was inevitable; in the same wards I was depressed by the thought that 40 per cent of babies with infantile diarrhoea were beyond my puny efforts; and these are but a few examples of our powerlessness less than forty years ago. But things have changed, and this is not due so much to the injection of money into the Health Service or to improved nutrition as to advances through medical research. Thus the introduction of the sulphonamides, penicillin, streptomycin, and their successors, has accomplished a major revolution in medical care. It cannot be denied that these improvements cost money but it would be difficult to imagine our financial problems in hospitals today if they had not occurred when they did. If the wards of our acute hospitals in 1977 continued to be filled with patients with infectious disease without effective chemotherapy, it would have been impossible to cope with patients who are now restored to good-quality life by joint replacement and by today's management of the now curable blood cancers. I suggest that this is a part of medical history which we should not forget because it will repeat itself and, through medical science, we will eventually get the results which society expects and to which it is entitled.

While a supporter of the view that well-planned health services research can, in the years ahead, result in a great improvement in the delivery of health care I consider that the future of the health service economy is closely bound up with the future of medical science and technology. It is probable that many secretly accept this view of the future while voicing the popular opinion that science, including medical science, is pricing itself out of the market and that each new discovery results in instruments or drugs of such complexity and excessive cost that science will wreck the national economy; precisely the opposite is my own belief. However, to believe is not enough. There is a need for an improved assessment of technology in the health industry as has become a routine and profitable exercise for other large industrial enterprises in this country. An inventory of our information, our methods, and a realistic prospect for the future is mandatory. Health and medicine has not been exposed sufficiently to this form of scrutiny. It would be easier to work out future policies, set future objectives, and make financial allocations if we had some system in operation to inform us, at any point in time, where we stand with technology, the cost of these measures, and whether considered options are likely to be affected by new or impending information. I imagine that engineers study likely future transport requirements before building new bridges so that their product will meet foreseeable demands and stresses; in medicine, we have permitted the development of artificial organs without counting the cost and this is surely a defect in our system—if we can claim to have a system. The explanation is to be found in history.

The profession of medicine stretches back over a thousand years or more during which dependence was placed on pseudo-technologies without science. Our patients expected the doctor to do something and so we undertook bleeding, purging, and the administration of methylene blue to mask the colour of haematuria; we still have our equivalents in medical practice all around us today. But science has now penetrated to the core of medicine and we must take a totally new look and organize our efforts. I am in agreement with Professor Thomas (34):

From now on, we will need, as never before, to keep the three central enterprises of medicine—to cure, to relieve, to comfort—clearly separated from each other in our minds. They do not really overlap, but we tend to view them, and the public takes the same view of course, as though they were all of a piece, all of the same body of technology, all derived from science, all modern. We try, consciously, or unconsciously, to pretend that there is more continuity than is really there, that everything we do is directed towards the same end. In fact, in real life, we are engaged in three entirely different kinds of technology in medicine. I have an idea that if we could conduct a sort of technology assessment on ourselves, and come to some sort of general agreement about which technology belongs in what category, we might be in a better position to make intelligent plans and forecast for the future, and we would almost surely be clearer in our minds about how to set priorities for the investment of scientific resources for the future.

He goes on to express an optimism which I share, namely, that the objective of controlling or eliminating disease is neither unthinkable nor beyond our imagining. In stating this belief I would emphasize that I make a distinction between ill health and human happiness, because the latter is quite a different matter and by no means the total responsibility of medicine and its practitioners. Like Shelley I can envisage disease being conquered, but I do not expect us to live for ever; it seems to me more likely that we are programmed to live for a predetermined life span but surely it is desirable to try to ensure that our span is characterized by good health. I will not enter here into the debate concerning the dangers of over-population; I would prefer over population with healthy individuals to over population with individuals requiring symptomatic treatment for chronic disease. It lies within our capacity to improve steadily the quality of life.

We are approaching the time when some of the most sought after treasures of the biological revolution will be made available to mankind. The molecular biologist now possesses instruments of immense power and he is exploring some of the most fundamental processes of life. While many regard medicine in our time as highly sophisticated, those favoured to glance back from the beginning of the twenty-first century will surely regard present practice as relatively primitive. Our present ignorance of the mechanisms of disease will be replaced by a fuller understanding of causation and this in turn will lead to effective treatment. The time for the application of medical science on a major scale is approaching and should not be hindered; medical practice will be totally transformed when it happens. However, in the immediate future we have no alternative but to face up to setting priorities and to making difficult choices between options and, in doing so, we must not lose sight of the fact that the practical application of existing scientific knowledge has not yet benefited more than a minority of earth's population. It is obligatory, as never before, to select between alternative possibilities in technology; we will require to make predictions concerning the outcome of different courses of action; as with all other great national enterprises, we are forced into the arena of technology assessment. Thomas (34) has described three different levels of technology in medicine and, persuaded by the arguments he presented in his lecture to the American College of Surgeons in 1974, I will draw unashamedly from his address in a consideration of the impacts of technology on medicine.

The first level to be considered can be called the 'high technology' of medicine. Its successes are decisive, lead to an understanding of the causation of a disease, and provide us with the capacity to deal with it effectively. My list of existing gains would include the use of antibiotics for bacterial infections, the prevention of haemolytic disease of the newborn, the treatment of endocrine disorders with appropriate hormones, etc., but I would have to agree with McKeown that the list is not yet extensive; I differ from him in my expectation that the turn of the century will see the list grow apace. The great advantage of high technology is that once knowledge is gained concerning the cause and treatment of a disease it is relatively inexpensive, relatively simple, and relatively easy to deliver. This message must be communicated convincingly if the support for research and training in the biomedical sciences is not to be allowed to decline.

I have earlier referred to the second level of medical technology, namely, 'halfway technology'. This represents the things we do, with varying success, to minimize the disability and suffering caused by a disease about which we have insufficient knowledge. Examples which come immediately to mind are transplantation of diseased organs, the use of cardiac bypass to permit the replacement of diseased valves and the introduction of an improved blood supply to the ischaemic heart, and the spectacular invention of artificial organs. The impending introduction of an artificial heart illustrates the nature of the dilemma which faces us as a result of the present emphasis on this level of technology. Despite the research effort currently made on a fuller understanding of cardiovascular disease it has to be admitted that there is, as yet, no real breakthrough. To regard the problem as insoluble in terms of understanding causative mechanisms would perhaps be a justification for letting the disease run its course until the organ is beyond repair, and then to introduce into the chest a nuclear-powered engine. If this approach is adopted I would have grave doubts about our ability to solve the problems of cost, distribution, and priority. The same sort of technology is at present being applied in the management of malignant disease in which we use surgery, radiotherapy, and chemical therapy when the disease is already well established; surely it is mandatory that we direct the main effort to an understanding of why a cell undergoes neoplastic change? There are those who believe that enough is already known to cope with this and other disease problems by the application of existing knowledge and that this approach should be given the highest priority. There are others (and I must place myself in this group) who believe that heart disease, cancer, and other killing diseases are soluble problems, given high-quality research by imaginative investigators. Which path do we take? We cannot afford both. It is characteristic of halfway technology that it is enormously expensive, requiring not only sophisticated equipment but highly trained staff to work it. It is of course difficult for doctors, and for society, to withhold a product of this kind of technology if it helps even a few patients and if it adds even a little to life expectancy or life quality. I can think of no acceptable way of reducing halfway technology other than by seeking new knowledge, and this can only come through good research.

The third level of technology, which Thomas (34) calls 'non-technology', is the substitute used by the medical profession when there is no means of altering the natural course or outcome of a disease process. It is sometimes referred to as 'supportive therapy' or 'caring', and so it is not a technology in any real sense but it is absolutely indispensible and every good doctor will spend much of his time in this aspect of his daily work. He did this for his patients with diphtheria, tuberculous meningitis, poliomyelitis, and the other infections which are now largely under control. The cost of this non-technology is very high and rises constantly.

It requires not only a great deal of time but also very hard effort and skill on the part of the physicians; only the very best of doctors are good at coping with this kind of defeat. It also involves long periods of hospitalisation, lots of nursing, lots of involvement of non-medical professionals in and out of the hospital. It represents, in short, a substantial segment of today's expenditures for health. It is not as great a financial problem for the future as halfway technology; but, between them, non-technology and halfway technology will sooner or later drive any system of health care that we may devise into bankruptcy.

Those responsible for the formulation of health policy, and who are presumably interested in saving money for health care in the long term, should consider that it would be an act of prudence to give high priority for the greater support of the health sciences. This is the surest way to rid ourselves of present dilemmas.

Because it is a live issue, it would be difficult to conclude without a comment on the organization and planning of medical research which has immediate implications for national science policy and for national health policy. Government calls for more applied research and development, more targeted research, more mission-orientated science and, at least by inference, less basic research. With something almost approaching confidence, this is associated with a demand for a new form of business orientated management which we are assured will allow us to reach our targets more quickly and more frugally. This drift gained momentum with the White Paper of 1972 which included the encouraging words that 'the new framework provides a partnership within which science will have more influence on the Government's central policy-making activities than before . . .'. If this hope can be realized, my optimism for the future would become even greater.

I have written at some length about my hopes for the growth of good health services research and indicated my confidence that this can result in significant improvements in the delivery of health care. I believe that this view is compatible with my avowed support for basic research in the biological sciences: they should run in tandem and a balance must be preserved.

It must be recognized that more applied science is not merely there for the asking. It may be relatively easy to obtain in areas such as defence but it is naive to think that it applies so readily to biology and medicine—a view which attributes to biology a much greater amount of usable information than is immediately available. It could be that we are close to developing sound applied science and the important decision to be made is whether this should be allowed to occur gradually as opportunity presents or whether it should (or can) be ordered more quickly by the injection of more money and new management. Of some things I am certain: the organization of research to improve the health service should avoid complexity and ensure flexibility; it must, without delay, find a mechanism for close and fruitful collaboration with the research councils; the research manager, the policymaker, and the scientist must be in the closest possible communication with each other; we must focus only on those problems for which the basic hard knowledge is available so that there is a high degree of certainty about a successful outcome from the beginning. In relation to the last, it is not difficult for the health departments to produce an extensive list of health problems but I know that an analysis of this list would yield a much smaller number of good questions for which the answers could be assured at this time. Nevertheless, we must try to extract these good questions and the logic of operational research should be invaluable in this exercise. I know that there would be much debate among the experts on priorities and on which questions are amenable to solution in the short term; perhaps the intensity and duration of debate could be used as a measure of the degree of certainty of gaining an answer! However we can have confidence that once the best set of questions based on hard knowledge has been agreed, these can be well studied by the most systematic methods of applied science. But let us be absolutely clear about the limitations of present knowledge and of the fact that we are not yet ready for full-scale applied science across the spectrum of disease problems: to decide on this approach now would slow down real progress or even bring it to a halt. If we continue to accumulate information of the power now being gained we will uncover the mechanisms of disease as we go along. I am optimistic enough to believe that, sooner or later, this will happen. What seemed to be insoluble problems a mere decade ago are now approachable, and the solution of some of them is discernible. It is only a matter of time.

> Our children's children shall see this, and bless heaven.
>
> Shakespeare, *Henry VIII*, Act v, scene v.

REFERENCES

1. *Memorandum on the Provisions of the Ministry of Health Bill, as to the work of the Medical Research Committee,* Cmnd 69 (1919).
2. HIMSWORTH, H. (1962). 'Society and the advancement of natural knowledge', *Br. med. J.* (15 December), 1537–63.
3. COHEN, R. H. L. (1973). In McLachlan, G. (ed.), *Portfolio for Health, 2, Problems and Progress in Medical Care,* Eighth Series (Oxford University Press for the Nuffield Provincial Hospitals Trust).
4. TOWNSEND, R. (1970). *Up the Organisation* (London: Michael Joseph).
5. WILDAVASKY, A. (1977). *Daedalus,* **26,** no. 1, pp. 105–23 (Cambridge, Mass.).
6. MUSTARD, J. F. (1977). 'Public policy and the future of Canadian health research', Address to the Canadian Society for Clinical Investigation (in press).
7. ROYAL COMMISSION ON MEDICAL EDUCATION (1968). *Report, 1965–68,* Cmnd 3569 (London: HMSO).
8. ASHBY, E. (1958). *Technology and the Academics* (London: Macmillan).
9. WHITEHEAD, A. N. (1976). *Science and the Modern World,* p. 248 (Cambridge: University Press).
10. PEART, W. S. (1973). 'Medical research is too important too be left to the researchers!', Lecture to mark the 25th anniversary of the foundation of the Glaxo Volume (Lilley, G. [ed.], vol. 38) (Glaxo Labs. Ltd).
11. DUNPHY, J. E. (1976). 'On caring for the patient with cancer', *Bull. Am. Coll. Surgeons,* **61,** 7.
12. MCCORMICK, R. A. (1975). 'The Karen Ann Quinlan case', *J. Am. Med. Ass.* **234,** 1057–8.
13. BROWN, JOHN (1900). 'Lectures on health', *Horae Subsecivae,* vol. 1 (London: Adam and Charles Black).
14. MCLACHLAN, G. (ed.) (1971). *In Low Gear? An Examination of 'Cogwheels'* (Oxford University Press for the Nuffield Provincial Hospitals Trust).
15. LEVITT, S., and GALLACHER, N. G. (1959). 'Prevention of venous thrombosis and pulmonary embolism in injured patients', *Lancet,* **ii,** 981–9.
16. MITCHELL, J. R. A. (1976). Addendum to Cochrane, A. L., 'Some reflections', in McLachlan, G. (ed.), *A Question of Quality?* (Oxford University Press for the Nuffield Provincial Hospitals Trust).

17. HIATT, H. H. (1973). 'Directions for research in the academic health centre', *J. med. Educ.* **48,** 55.

18. WANGENSTEEN, S. L. *et al.* (1959). 'Depressant action of local gastric hypothermia on gastric digestion', *J. Am. Med. Ass.* **169,** 1601.

19. COX, A. G. *et al.* (1968). *GUT,* **9,** 411.

20. WILSON, G. M. (1976). 'The Hospital Health Services Research Unit', in McLachlan, G. (ed.), *A Question of Quality?* (Oxford University Press for the Nuffield Provincial Hospitals Trust).

21. KAY, A. W. (1976). Screening for colon cancer', *Health Bulletin,* **34,** 347–54.

22. BLACK, J. W. *et al.* (1972). *Nature, Lond.* **236,** 385.

23. HARRIS, H. (1974). *Prenatal Diagnosis and Selective Abortion,* Rock Carling Monograph (London: Nuffield Provincial Hospitals Trust).

24. FERGUSON-SMITH, M. A. (1974), 'Prenatal diagnosis', *The Practitioner,* **213,** 655.

25. WADDINGTON, C. H. (1973). In Introduction to 'Advances in molecular genetics', *Br. med. Bull.* **29,** 185–7.

26. BRENNER, S. (1975). 'Genetics of behaviour', ibid. **29,** 269–71.

27. *Report of the Working Party on the Experimental Manipulation of the Genetic Composition of Micro-organisms* (Chairman: Lord Ashby), Cmnd 5880 (London: HMSO).

28. ZIFF, E. (1973). 'Benefits and hazards of manipulating DNA', *New Scientist,* **60,** 274–5.

29. HIGGINS, I. T. T. (1975). 'Epidemiological studies', *Br. med. Bull.* **31,** 230–5.

30. NEUBERGER, A. (1975). In Introduction to 'Chemicals in food and environment', ibid. **31,** 181–3.

31. DOLL, R. (1973). *Medicine in the 21st Century,* International Symposium to celebrate the Centenary of the Manchester Medical School (Manchester: Geigy).

32. DOLL, R. (1967). *Prevention of Cancer: Pointers from Epidemiology,* Rock Carling Monograph (London: Nuffield Provincial Hospitals Trust).

33. MCKEOWN, T. (1976). *The Role of Medicine: Dream, Mirage, or Nemesis?,* Rock Carling Monograph (London: Nuffield Provincial Hospitals Trust).

34. THOMAS, L. (1974). 'The future impact of science and technology on medicine', *Bull. Am. Coll. Surgeons,* **59,** no. 6, 25.

In addition, much help was gained from the following:

BLACK, SIR DOUGLAS (1972). 'Rothschild and medical research', *Lancet,* **i,** 254.

COCHRANE, A. L. (1972). *Effectiveness and Efficiency,* Rock Carling Monograph (London: Nuffield Provincial Hospitals Trust).

References

Dunlop, G. R. (1976). 'Medical costs—our common dilemma', *Bull. Am. Coll. Surgeons,* **61,** no. 11, 7–11.

Fletcher, C. M. (1972). *Communication in Medicine*, Rock Carling Monograph (London: Nuffield Provincial Hospitals Trust).

Halpert, H. P. (1973). 'Research utilization, a problem in goal setting: what is the question?', *Am. J. Publ. Hlth,* **63,** 377.

Heard, A. (1976). 'Public policy and the paradoxes of plenty', *Bull. Am. Coll. Surgeons,* **61,** no. 12, 9–15.

Himsworth, H. (1970). *The Development and Organization of Scientific Knowledge* (London: Heinemann).

Kass, E. H. (1973). 'Biomedical research opportunities in the health maintenance organisation', *J. med. Educ.* **48,** no. 4, 103.

McMichael, J. (1973). 'Research and understanding', *Postgrad. med. J.* **49,** 441–5.

Zuckerman, Sir Solly (1970). *Beyond the Ivory Tower* (London: Weidenfeld and Nicolson).